Tourism and Maternal Health

Anthropology of Well-Being

Individual, Community, Society

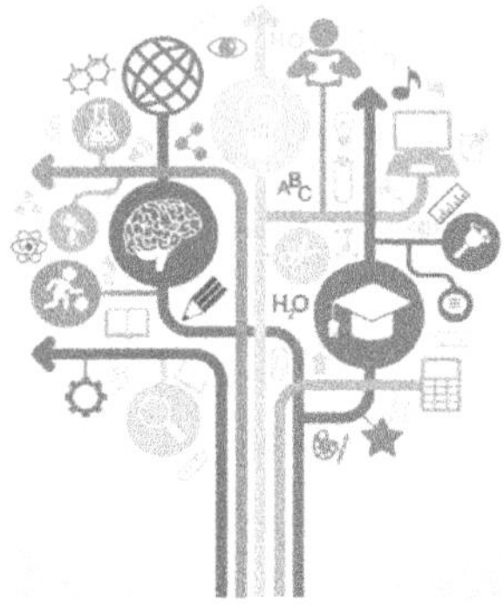

Series Editor: Ben G. Blount, PhD (SocioEcological Informatics)

Mission Statement

Well-being is central and important in people's daily lives and life history. This book series brings about understanding of what the complex concepts of well-being include. The concepts of quality of life, life satisfaction, and happiness will be explored and viewed at the individual level, the community level, and the level of society. The series encourages and promotes research into the concept of well-being, how it appears to be defined culturally, and how it is utilized across levels and across different social, economic, and ethnic groups. Understandings of how well-being promotes stability and resilience will also be critical to advances in understanding, as well as how well-being can be implemented as a goal in resisting vulnerabilities and in adaptation. Series books include monographs and edited collections by a range of academics, from rising scholars to experts in relevant fields.

Advisory Board Members

Books in Series

Tourism and Maternal Health: Customs, Beliefs, and Everyday Practices, by Allison R. Cantor

Contesting Pharmaceuticals: Production, Circulation, Uses of the Material Objects of Therapies by Pino Schirippa, translated by Ciaran Durkan

Well-Being as a Multidimensional Concept: Understanding Connections among Culture, Community, and Health, edited by Janet M. Page-Reeves

Romantic Love in America: Cultural Models of Gay, Straight, and Polyamorous Relationships, by Victor C. de Munck

Three Fruits: Nepali Ayurvedic Doctors on Health, Nature, and Social Change, by Mary M. Cameron

Black Women and Breast Cancer: A Cultural Theology, by Elizabeth A. Williams

Cultural Dimensions of Well-Being: Therapy Animals as Healers, by Clementine K. Fujimura and Simone Nommensen

Love in the Time of Ethnography edited by Lucinda Carspecken

Contemporary Conversations on Immigration in the United States: The View from Prince George's County, Maryland, by Judith Noemí Freidenberg

Intimate Partner Violence and Advocate Response: Redefining Love in Western Belize by Melissa Beske

Tourism and Maternal Health

Customs, Beliefs, and Everyday Practices

Allison R. Cantor

LEXINGTON BOOKS
Lanham • Boulder • New York • London

Published by Lexington Books
An imprint of The Rowman & Littlefield Publishing Group, Inc.
4501 Forbes Boulevard, Suite 200, Lanham, Maryland 20706
www.rowman.com

6 Tinworth Street, London SE11 5AL, United Kingdom

British Library Cataloguing in Publication Information Available

Library of Congress Control Number: 2019949529

ISBN: 978-1-7936-0425-5 (cloth : alk. paper)
ISBN: 978-1-7936-0426-2 (electronic)

For Renee and Marvin.

Contents

List of Figures and Tables

FIGURES

TABLES

Acknowledgments

First and foremost, thank you to all of the women in the Monteverde Zone for your friendship while I conducted the research presented in this book. It would not have been possible without you. The support of the Monteverde Institute was instrumental in bringing this work to fruition; the never-ending supply of coffee and laughter kept me going when I thought I would never finish. I would also like to thank Nancy Romero-Daza and David Himmelgreen. I could never have imagined how far my academic career would take me when I met you in Monteverde all those years ago. Thank you for the continued support, friendship, and constructive criticism. I truly would not be here without you. Thank you. Thank you, Daniel Lende for your mentorship. Rita DeBate, thank you for your input on the original research from the public health perspective and helping me to understand the realities of doing health-related research, which didn't always fit with my own ideas. And thank you, Barbara Piperata for your thoughtful, insightful, and honest critique of the dissertation on which this manuscript is based. Thank you, Jenny Peña, for being a constant source of friendship and guidance and reminding me that I was gaining local insight during the literal and figurative *aguaceros* I experienced over the years. I also want to thank my mom, dad, and sister for their overwhelming love and support. Thank you to my husband. I know that being away from family, friends, and *chile* was a sacrifice for you. Thank you for your input on earlier versions of the manuscript and for keeping me in check. Thank you, Sebastian for putting up with my many hours of writing and for being my inspiration. I would also like to thank the University of South Florida's College of Public Health and the Department of Anthropology for awarding me a research scholarship and the Dissertation Completion Fellowship, which allowed me to complete the research for this manuscript.

Introduction

The thick white clouds rolled across the narrow and rocky dirt road. The air was sweet and heavy and smelled like the earth after a long rain. The clouds bathed the green tropical forest that seemed to spill onto the sides of the passage. The laconic call of the bellbird, one of Monteverde's[1] most iconic species, seemed to come from every direction. Its terse song complemented the sounds of the morning, which included other birds, dairy cattle moving from one pasture to the next, and the constant buzz of machinery coming from the Monteverde Cheese Factory. The road appeared deserted and left me feeling as though I was the only one wandering this tropical landscape. And then, I heard the sound of the out-of-commission yellow school bus coming around the bend, bringing tourists to the Monteverde Cloud Forest Reserve. The bus was full and was followed by a large tank truck that read, *transporta leche* (milk transport). I was quickly reminded that this isolated tropical paradise was not "isolated," but was connected with the global market economy through tourism and the presence of the Mexican conglomerate, Sigma, which purchased the Monteverde Cheese Factory in 2013 (Sigma Alimentos 2013). These two economic activities meant that there was a constant flux of people and goods in and out of this rural mountain region. This observation exemplifies the inherent contradictions that exist in the rural highlands of Costa Rica, and elsewhere, as local systems grapple with an increasingly global society. One in which a seemingly sleepy rural region with 6,000 local residents now hosts over 250,000[2] tourists annually (Hamilton 2015).

On my first trip to the Monteverde Zone in 2008, I was struck by the paradoxes I saw within the local food system. For example, there was a "local" farmer's market that only had a few producers from the surrounding area, and while there were no fast food chain restaurants, there were more pizza joints than were necessary for a small rural community. Perhaps the most surprising tension existed in the relationship between food insecurity and tourism. In one of the top tourist destinations in Costa Rica, many local people were suffering from the effects of food insecurity, defined by the World Health Organization (2016a) as, "lack of access to sufficient, safe, nutritious food to maintain a healthy and active life." As my background is in maternal and child health, this led me to wonder how pregnant women were faring in this economically rich, yet nutritionally poor environment. Over time, I realized that the tension was perhaps greatest for pregnant women, who were bound by social practices regarding the perinatal period, such as *cuarentena,* a postpartum time of rest, but who were also engaging in modern lifestyles as a result of rapid growth and development in the region (Cantor et al. 2013). Early on in my research, I was asked to give a talk on nutrition at a local birth class. The red soda fizzed and bubbled like champagne in the small clear plastic cups. As one nurse walked around to serve soda from the cafeteria trays, another handed out small Styrofoam plates with two half sandwiches and two small marmalade-filled cookies to pregnant women participating in the preparation for birth course at the clinic. I took a bite of what I thought was a mustard and cheese sandwich. It was actually *Numar*, a popular margarine made from hydrogenated oil. It was caked on as thick as mustard and overpowered the thin slice of Bimbo-brand processed white bread. I examined the other half sandwich, but only after taking a bite did I determine that it was mostly mayonnaise with oily canned tuna fish, dotted with chopped vegetables. I watched as another tray came around with watermelon and I heard the nurses urging women to take more than one slice, one for them and one for the baby. I was scheduled to give a talk on nutrition to this group of pregnant women and their partners, although I was unsure how to proceed, as the snack being served had the sugars, fats, processed foods, and portion sizes that I was about to critique. I looked around to see how the women were reacting. Some sat smiling and quietly ate with their partners. A few gave questioning looks at what they were being served but ate it anyway, and some discretely poured the soda out in the bathroom sink. This example highlights the complex ways that humans interact with and react to the environment around them, including the food landscape. So what happens when the food environment rapidly shifts and there is a transition from an agricultural-based subsistence lifestyle to one based on tourism? What are the impacts on maternal health in this context?

The purpose of this book is to address these questions using formal research conducted from June 2014 to August 2015, while drawing on collective participant observation experiences since 2008. This book examines how prenatal dietary practices have shifted over time in the face of rapid tourism-driven growth and development in the Monteverde Zone and explores how pregnant women today make decisions about their own dietary behaviors.

This book focuses on the links between tourism, the nutrition transition (Popkin and Reardon 2018), and prenatal diet. While there is abundant literature on the nutrition transition as a conceptual and analytical framework (Popkin 2017; Parra et al. 2015; Jayawardena et al. 2017; Kraft et al. 2018), little work has been conducted to date on the ways that the nutrition transition influences prenatal dietary practices and nutritional status. While there are some notable studies (Kavle et al. 2017; Giordano and Benyshek 2015; Abu-Saad et al. 2012), this book fills the gap in the literature.

A main argument of this book is that in order to understand how large shifts in our nutritional environment affect actual dietary practices and nutritional status, in-depth studies need to be conducted to identify which aspects of the human condition allow us to successfully (or unsuccessfully) adapt and cope with nutritional stress. The overall goal of this book is to provide an in-depth account of the ways in which pregnant women interact with the Monteverde Zone's rapidly changing food landscape, and in doing so, contribute to the literature on the nutrition transition (Popkin 2017) and the critical biocultural approach (CBCA) (Leatherman and Goodman 2011).

In the following pages, I will show how various aspects of culture protect pregnant women from the negative health impacts of the tourism industry, while highlighting the complex process through which changes in the food environment impact women's decision-making. Just as the women in the birth class were given contradictory information (between the lecture on nutrition and a meal that spoke to opposite behaviors), women in the Monteverde Zone are faced with these types of situations everyday, forcing them to make decisions about their own prenatal health. This work contributes to case studies in global health by revealing the processes through which culturally situated decision-making about health behaviors change over time. This book also has implications for evidence-based strategies to prevent and alleviate food insecurity and malnutrition.

This book examines the role of the tourism-driven nutrition transition in shaping prenatal dietary practices and identifies key aspects of the relationship between the shifting food environment and prenatal food insecurity in this region. Food insecurity during pregnancy can affect weight gain, increase the risks for pregnancy complications, and contribute to psychosocial stress (Laraia et al. 2010, 2006). This not only affects individual health and well-being, but also has the potential to impact families, communities, and nations.

RESEARCH DESIGN

The bulk of this book is based on field research conducted from 2014 to 2015. In order to complete the ethnographic picture presented here, I also drew on field experiences beginning in 2008. During that year, I lived with a family in the Monteverde Zone for a little over a month while I participated in a community health field program. This was the first time my ethnographic mind was engaged in a real field setting. I returned in 2009 as a research affiliate at the Monteverde Institute to conduct an individual research project on prenatal nutrition in the context of globalization. Subsequently, I visited during the summer months of 2011 and 2012 to reconnect with study participants, my affiliate organization, and other friends. As a doctoral student, I was lucky enough to work at my field site in an official capacity, as a course assistant for a National Science Foundation-funded research experience for undergraduates for three years during the summer months of 2013, 2014, and 2015, which overlapped with my formal field research. This gave me the opportunity to actively engage with methods in community health research (through teaching, advising undergraduates, and research) and to build rapport with local entities, such as the clinic and the municipality. In 2015, I started teaching for the Monteverde Institute, which allowed me to bring my experience with community-engaged research into the classroom through an experiential learning curriculum.

Throughout my time spent in the Monteverde Zone, I learned to do community-based research. However, one doesn't "do" community-based research but learns to engage in the process of working in communities. The amalgamation of my experiences in this community led to a research design that was appropriate for this setting. Many people in the community knew who I was or were familiar with my past work in the area, which allowed me to build rapport easily and provided me access to certain spaces, such as the preparation for birth class at the local clinic. Further, my own familiarity with the ethnographic realities of working in the area (e.g., the Costa Rica cultural conception of time) permitted me to design a study that was realistic and feasible. This also helped with the analysis of data (e.g., creating conceptual categories from free listing data), as I have established a solid foundation of cultural knowledge over time that has provided insight to the emic (i.e., insider's) perspective regarding the topic of food and nutrition. It's also important to note that my strong relationship with the Monteverde Institute and the community health program meant that the head of this department, a Costa Rican and long-time resident of the zone, was instrumental in making sure the research was ethical and appropriate for this community context.

Overall, I conducted forty-two semi-structured interviews with a convenience sample of mothers in the region. Twenty-two of these women were pregnant at the time of the interview and also participated in dietary recalls and a food insecurity questionnaire. I administered fifty-two street-intercept surveys with a random sample of men and women from the community, which also included various free listing exercises. I held two participatory focus groups with mothers from different communities. These were completed early on in the research process in order to give context to the rest of the research.

Ethics

The small population of the region, approximately 6,000 residents, created an environment in which most individuals were connected to others through familial ties, social ties, or by the sheer fact that they had been residents of the Monteverde Zone for so long that they had crossed paths at one time or another. This was a delicate situation when I conducted interviews, as there are no street addresses in the Monteverde Zone and therefore the taxi drivers needed to know the name of the individual or the family name of the individual in order to get me where I needed to go. Additionally, due to the limited number of taxi drivers in town, many knew me and knew about my research. In order to address this, I tried to work with the same driver who I trusted and who assured me he would maintain confidentiality regarding the women I would visit. However, once, as we pulled up to a farmhouse that was twenty minutes outside of town, the driver wanted to say hello to my participant, as she was a good friend of his mother's. We walked up to the house and my participant's niece was in the kitchen cooking. She explained that her aunt would be back in a few minutes, as she was out picking limes. When she finally arrived she was wearing dirty jeans and black rubber work boots, and this sixty-year-old woman was carrying a sack of limes over her back that rivaled her own stature. She greeted us and invited both of us to breakfast. We chatted and ate a typical Costa Rican breakfast together. When we were done, she walked me out back so we could have some privacy and conduct our interview. After the interview. the three of us walked around her property and she showed us all the food she was growing. This was a typical scene for this small town, and it could not be avoided, as the social fabric of the community dictated that you be flexible with time (sometimes referred to as *Tico* time[3]) (*Tico*[4] is the self-described name for Costa Ricans) and that you always engage in social activities when the opportunities presented themselves. Additionally, the free listing activity was conducted on the street in the center of town and it is possible that others in the community saw someone they knew participating in my study. Despite situations like these, I did not disclose to taxi drivers or other individuals who my participants were and did not share participants' personal information.[5] Participant compensation was a major ethical concern in research design. Since giving participants cash may have created unnecessary bias in this sample, I gave each participant a gift for his or her time.[6]

Additionally, there are certain ethical and political dimensions to consider when conducting in-depth ethnographic research (Christians 2011), as lines often become blurred between "research" and personal relationships, especially during participant observation (Angrosino and Rosenberg 2011). As I became close with some participants who I would see frequently around town or visit after the data collection had ended, it became difficult to separate myself from my role as a researcher, as I was always observing the environment around me for clues to better understand the cultural construction of diet within this sociocultural context. In order to address this, I always made sure to talk about my work as a subtle reminder to them that I was interested in food-related behaviors, even outside of the formal data collection phase that they participated in.

Positionality

"The notion of positionality rests on the assumption that a culture is more than a monolithic entity to which one belongs or not" (Merriam et al. 2001, 411). As Merriam and colleagues (2001) point out, the line between insider and outsider is often blurry at best, as these identity categories are not easily defined within sociocultural spaces that inherently have internal variation. It is important to reflect on positionality here, as my identity within the Monteverde Zone ultimately shaped my research design and implementation. It is important to reflect on my own role within the community since it impacted the way that participants (and potential participants) interacted with me and perceived my work. This ultimately affected specific elements of the research design. As I see it, I wear three different hats in the Monteverde Zone. For those I have come to know well over the years, I am a friend and recurrent visitor. I am also a research affiliate and seasonal employee at local nonprofit organization, which connects me politically and professionally to a specific faction of the community. Finally, to everyone else I am an outsider and a tourist. What this third distinction means is that people in the zone charge me more for food, housing, and transportation than locals and constantly try to get me to buy their products and use their services (e.g., taxis, tours, and hotels). I am not denying that I am a tourist. On the contrary, I recognize that I am a tourist, a visitor, and a guest in this community. My different roles within the Monteverde Zone and my long-standing relationship with the community affected this study in two important ways. First, my experience living and working in the region for over twenty months between 2008 and 2015 allowed me to access the community in ways that those unfamiliar with the region or the people would not have been able to. Second, my role as a tourist or outsider was valuable in helping me to apply the etic (i.e., outsider's) perspective to analyzing the ways that larger explanatory frameworks (e.g., the nutrition transition and the CBCA) play out within this local context.

However, my role as an outsider also provided certain challenges throughout this investigation. I was unable to get the overall ethnographic depth that I had originally planned to because of the historical relationship between locals, tourists, and researchers. I did learn a lot about these relationships, although many of the details are beyond the scope of this work. I learned about decision-making and dietary practices from my participants' narratives, which were supplemented with participant observation that I engaged in everyday through community events, time with my Tico friends, volunteer work, and employment at a local institution. This role as an outsider did allow me to ask obvious questions and probe about taken-for-granted aspects of life, which would have seemed out of place to those that consider themselves my friends in the Monteverde Zone. This challenge altered the research design (i.e., using narrative to understand food-related practices as opposed to firsthand observation and the inability to explore, in depth, how women actually behaved in various social situations) and may partially account for the low sample size of (n=42). However, this experience also reflects the realities in practicing ethnography in an environment that has been saturated by researchers and outsiders.

All participant names presented in this book are pseudonyms. The name of my affiliate organization and the communities are not hidden, as this area has been the focal point of many research endeavors and it would be very obvious which region I am referring to as I provide historical context for the work presented here. In addition, I hope to contribute to studies in global health and promote international partnerships. By the transparency presented here, readers can see what local organizations are doing to engage with community health in this increasingly global age.

CHAPTER ORGANIZATION

In chapters 1 (The Monteverde Zone) and 2 (Tourism), I set the contextual setting for the research presented in this book. The Monteverde Zone is a rural area in the Costa Rican highlands with a reputation for ecotourism. This makes the region a good place to start when examining the impacts of rapidly shifting foodways on maternal health, as the tourism boom in the 1990s has led to dramatic changes in lifestyle in a short amount of time (at least at the time the data was collected for this book in 2014–2015). These chapters describe the history of the Monteverde Zone and the role that tourism has played in shaping various aspects of community life, including health.

In chapter 3 (The Nutrition Transition), I outline the nutrition transition (Popkin 2012). I use this overarching framework to explain the relationship between global development and contemporary health issues, such as the rise in chronic noncommunicable disease. I argue that a tourism-driven nutrition transition has occurred in the Monteverde Zone and may play a role in shaping the health trends previously documented in the region (Cantor et al. 2013; Himmelgreen et al. 2006, 2014). However, there are many critiques of this framework as an explanatory model and in chapter 4 (Expanding the Nutrition Transition), I draw on the CBCA (Leatherman and Goodman 2011) and practice theory (Ortner 1997) to bridge the gaps in the nutrition transition model. Linking the CBCA with practice theory makes an important contribution to understanding how facets of global development, such as tourism, ultimately shape prenatal diet, nutrition, and health in a local context. In this chapter, I also identify various elements of praxis, which illuminate the important contributions of this text.

In chapter 5 (Customs), I show how culture still plays an important role in informing diet and nutrition, despite rapid changes to the local food environment. Customs, or *costumbres,* had a marked influence over dietary practices and culturally situated ideas about nutrition. This chapter outlines the ways in which nutrition is constructed as a local cultural process. Through triangulation of free listing data (n=52) with semi-structured interviews (n=42) and focus groups (N=2, n=15), I show how this construct is part of a shared national and regional identity.

In chapter 6 (Cultural Beliefs and Everyday Practices), I illustrate how collective ideas about what constitutes acceptable, or culturally appropriate prenatal dietary practices (i.e., dietary taboos, prescriptions, and cravings) are shared and ubiquitous. I also explain how cultural beliefs, or *creencias*, are deeply embedded in these shared dietary practices. This chapter reveals how ideas about normative behaviors shape health outcomes. Everyday practices, often described by women as *lo normal,* or "the usual," were consistently used to describe prenatal dietary practices among study participants and is reflected in actual consumption patterns. This chapter uses dietary intake data to show how the idea of consuming what is "normal" guided dietary practices and actual nutritional intake during the prenatal period.

In chapter 7 (Engaging in Practice: Decision-Making and Human Agency), I illustrate the ways that local belief systems influence decision-making for women during the perinatal period. Some beliefs are inextricably linked with women's attitudes toward food and nutrition and their own decision-making regarding dietary practices. Decision-making was also intertwined with food access, social actors, and the production of knowledge. In this chapter, I describe the relationship between decision-making and health, illustrating the ways that women's decision-making processes during pregnancy have changed over time in the context of tourism-related development.

In chapter 8 (Tourism and Culture Change), I describe the relationship between changing local customs and tourism, emphasizing the way that culture is changing in response to the transition to a tourism economy, which began a little over a generation ago. Most notably, These changes occur through various cultural influences and access to work opportunities. I also discuss food access in this context and describe prenatal food insecurity as it impacts the women in this book.

In the conclusion, I review the contribution that a practice-oriented approach makes to the CBCA in anthropology and the nutrition transition framework. This contribution to theory is useful in the context of expanding contemporary maternal health research, as this work is used to address the constantly changing global society that is also guided by traditional cultural norms and values. This explicitly shows how global development impacts maternal health and describes the implications of these relationships for public health and work in the social sciences.

NOTES

1. While pseudonyms are used for all study participants, the names of locations have only been altered in some cases, such as when referring to focus group communities. I decided to include the regional names for locations because this area is already well-known and well-studied in the context of the themes presented in this book.

2. Unfortunately, there is no centralized way to collect data on the number of tourists that travel to the Monteverde Zone. The estimate that 250,000 people visit the Monteverde annually comes from the director of the Monteverde Institute, Debra Hamilton, who has access to various sources of data that track the number of tourists at various locations, such as the Monteverde Cloud Forest Reserve.

3. "Tico time" refers to the different conceptualization of time that exists in Costa Rica. It is not uncommon for individuals or groups to show up fifteen to thirty minutes late to meetings or events, or for individuals to commit to do something "right now," which actually means sometime in the near future.

4. Costa Ricans are referred to as *Ticos*, as they often use their own form of the diminutive in their speech. For example, in place of saying *chiquito* (i.e., small) (without diminutive) or *chiquitito* (i.e., very small) (with the diminutive), they might say *chiquitico* (i.e., very small) (regional version of the diminutive).

5. All data were coded with a participant identification number and personal information was stored in a password-protected excel database, which included participants' names, identification number, and contact information. All other study data were stored in a password-protected database and de-identified to ensure participant anonymity. Participants were also given my contact information and the information for the Monteverde Institute so that they could contact me with further questions or comments.

6. Street-intercept participants received fruits from one of the local grocery stores or farmer's market worth $5 (2,669.08 Costa Rican colones). For all other participants, each gift was worth approximately $10 (5,315.80 Costa Rican colones). Pregnant women received something for their baby (e.g., clothes, baby shampoo, talcum powder, etc.) and older women received a scarf.

Chapter 1

The Monteverde Zone

Cow. This is the first word that comes to my mind when thinking about the Monteverde Zone. This region was home to such high dairy production that at one point it became known as the milkshed of Costa Rica. While "watershed" is the term typically used to describe an "area that channels rainfall and snowmelt to creeks, streams, and rivers, and eventually to outflow points such as reservoirs, bays, and the ocean" (NOAA 2018), "milkshed" describes the Monteverde Zone, since this region has produced milk for some of the top cheese producers in Costa Rica. Historically, dairy cows are a common sighting in the area, causing morning traffic jams and quietly and constantly grazing on green pastures lining unpaved roads. Throughout my many years of visiting, living, and working in this region, I came into close contact with dairy cattle. During the fieldwork for this book, I found myself alone, on a rural dirt road confronting a bovine specimen more than once. The first time, I was walking to an interview. I half focused on the road, as not to trip over any rocks or slip on gravel, and half prepared notes in my head. I was walking on a slight decline and as I peered over the crest of the road in front of me, I noticed a large dairy cow. She was staring at me, standing in the middle of the road. I was unsure what to do. Clearly, she was unsure what to do, as this dusty path was not her usual grazing area. I greeted the cow and she just stared. I stared back. As I started walking toward her, she backed off and turned down a side road. Another day, I was walking home from an interview in a community on the other side of town. I was thinking about the interview when I looked up to see a bull in the road, staring at me intently. There was barbwire fencing on both sides of the road and no obvious escape from this situation. I did not have cell service. The agitated bull started to snort. My heart raced. Suddenly, I heard what sounded like a cow from a nearby pasture. The bull turned its head and quickly jumped over one of the fences, disappearing from my sight. These experiences, which both occurred early on in my fieldwork, reminded me that despite the rise in tourism in this area and the ways that the Monteverde Zone was inextricably linked with the rest of the world through various global forces, this was still a rural region where one could, from time to time, find themselves alone on a dirt road with no cell service, an agitated bull, and nowhere to go.

REGIONAL CONTEXT: THE MONTEVERDE ZONE

The geographical area I have been referring to thus far is called, the "Monteverde Zone" and includes the district of Monte Verde (meaning "green mountain"), located in the county of Puntarenas in Puntarenas Province, one of the seven provinces that divide Costa Rica. However, depending on the context, the Monteverde Zone can include communities in the nearby counties of Tilarán and Abangares, which are located in the neighboring province of Guanacaste. Although Puntarenas and Guanacaste are typically perceived as representing different cultural and economic entities, the development of the Monteverde Zone as a noteworthy area with its own identity occurred in direct relationship to the economic activities that have historically defined this geographic space, which includes dairy farming and tourism (Vivanco 2006). Despite the fact that some communities in this region belong to different provinces, the development of the ecotourism industry has created a space that transcends political boundaries.

The Monteverde Zone is home to some of Costa Rica's cloud forest, which makes it a major tourist destination. The cloud forest ecosystem, also referred to as tropical montane cloud forest, is characterized by altitudinal range and the presence of clouds (continuous, seasonal, or persistent) which frequently envelope or pass through vegetation as a direct result of the altitude (Hamilton et al. 1995). The tropical montane cloud forest in the Americas accounts for 40.8 percent of this forest type, globally, and in general, this ecological niche is known for its high levels of biodiversity (Bruijnzeel et al. 2010). The Monteverde Cloud Forest reaches heights of 1,850 meters or 6,070 feet above sea level (Monteverde Cloud Forest Biological Reserve n.d.) and is located in the highlands of the Tilarán mountain range within the crux of the continental divide. The district of Monte Verde has approximately 4,155 residents (INEC 2011), most of which are centrally located in the town of Santa Elena (Ministerio de Salud 2015). However, it is difficult to calculate the actual population since the Monteverde Zone encompasses more than one province and local self-identification can be fluid. The resident population is comprised of Ticos, international residents, and Quaker descendants from the United States.

In the 1950s, North American Quakers settled in the township of Monteverde (Vivanco 2006) (located within the district of Monte Verde). This group has played a major role in the development of local conservation efforts, sustainable tourism, and the opening and continued presence of the Monteverde Cheese Factory. As a direct result of the growth and development of this particular region, there are also long and short-term international residents. Key features that guided development in the Monteverde Zone include an emphasis on sustainability and access to a unique ecological niche with extreme biodiversity that was ripe for research. Today, the community is also comprised of educators and students who come to teach at one of the area's two private K–12 schools, one of the local higher educational entities (e.g., the Monteverde Institute and the Council on International Educational Exchange), or who come with school groups participating in short- and long-term courses in and around the Monteverde Zone. Researchers from an array of disciplines, including environmental studies, biology, sustainability studies, history, sociology, and anthropology, are also drawn to this region and participate in a range of short-term or ongoing investigations. Additionally, there are artists and retirees who are originally from other regions in Latin America, North America, and other countries, such as Israel.

HISTORICAL CONTEXT: TICOS, QUAKERS, AND THE MILKSHED

In general, Costa Rica is not a destination for archaeology tourism. Some tourists assume that this is due to the lack of archaeology or indigenous culture in the country as a whole. Despite active efforts to present Ticos as a homogenous ethnicity, there are indigenous peoples in Costa Rica and their presence throughout the region should be acknowledged. Although the Monteverde Zone, along with other areas of Costa Rica, have been inhabited on and off since prehistoric times, there has been little research to date on the archaeological sites or the human material remains found in the area. Farmers commonly find artifacts in their fields and petroglyphs and potential burial sites have been described in the nearby forest. Additionally, local conservationists have identified a series of forest trails that lead to Arenal Volcano (approximately 85 miles away) (monteverdeinfo 2011) and have crossroads with other pathways. During a recent renovation of the area's main soccer plaza, an arrowhead was found that some believe could date back 8000–9000 years (Saenz 2015)[1]. Unlike some other areas of Costa Rica, there is no indication of indigenous culture today, although the presence of artifacts ties local Ticos to their regional history and contributes to identity, since locals take advantage of opportunities to learn about how to preserve artifacts and what to do when they find material remains on their property. Historical records show that the area was inhabited as early as 1902, and there were possibly indigenous peoples living in the region until 1910–1911 (Saenz 2015). In the 1920s and 1930s the government was pushing a manifest destiny type of policy to encourage Ticos to settle outside of the Central Valley (Saenz 2015). If they were willing to relocate, they were offered land. It was during this period that families began to settle in the area, many from San Ramón (halfway between the Monteverde Zone and San José, the country's capital), and they engaged in subsistence agriculture. Descendants of these families still live in the area today and many are community leaders and local business owners.

In the early 1950s a group of Quakers from the United States settled in what is now known as the town of Monteverde. Quakerism is a religion that was first founded in seventeenth-century England in response to Puritanism (Hamm 2004). Although the Quaker movement was unified at its inception, rifts in the 1820s led to the diversification of the originally Christian-based faith (Hamm 2004). However, some core tenets still characterize the Quaker religion as distinct, such as the consensus style decision-making, the value placed on education, and the dedication to pacifism (Hamm 2004). Due to their Quaker beliefs, four men from Alabama refused to register for the draft after the U.S. Military Training Act was passed in 1948 (Rockwell 2015). They were subsequently sentenced to prison for one year and one day, but they only served one-third of their sentence and thereafter decided to leave the United States. They were released on October 27, 1950, and left Fairhope, Alabama on November 4 for Costa Rica. At some points during their journey they had to make their own road, since the Pan-American Highway was not yet completed. Seven families were involved in the resettlement and members of their group previously travelled throughout Central America identifying Costa Rica as a good place to relocate to, especially since the country abolished its army in 1948 (Molina and Palmer 2007), which was in line with Quaker pacifism. They arrived on February 1, 1951, and rented apartments in San José while they looked for land to purchase. They knew they wanted to be at an altitude where malaria would not be a problem, and after viewing numerous properties, they decided on the Monteverde Zone. The Quakers decided to produce cheese as their major economic activity since cheese would stay fresh long enough for them to make the trek down the mountain to sell their product in the Central Valley (Rockwell 2015). In 1953, they opened the Monteverde Cheese Factory (Costa Rica Study Tours 2013). The business was formed as a cooperative and consensus style decision-making was used to make plans for the direction of the company, as this model fit within the ethical modality that characterizes Quakerism. This became a major economic driver in the region, causing many Ticos to adopt dairy farming. This region became known locally as the milkshed because of the amount of milk that was produced to support the activities at the Monteverde Cheese Factory, which included making cheese and ice cream. According to their website (2013), the Monteverde Cheese Factory was the first business in Monteverde, and the Quakers were the first to produce pasteurized cheese in Costa Rica. At the time the data was collected for this book, the Monteverde Cheese Factory was the second largest producer of cheese in Costa Rica. In 2013, Sigma, a Mexican conglomerate corporation, purchased the Monteverde Cheese Factory (Sigma Alimentos 2013) and has made many changes, although they still produce and sell some ice cream and cheese items, along with other Sigma products. The long-term impacts of this change have yet to be seen, although part of the original sale contract was that the factory would remain open in Monteverde for three years. Three years has passed, and although the Monteverde Cheese Factory is still open to tourists, they have discontinued their factory tour, closed their restaurant, and have ceased to produce several cheese products, such as *queso fresco* (i.e., farmer's cheese), which is now produced at another factory in the country and then shipped to the Monteverde Cheese Factory to sell. The Monteverde Cheese Factory also sells other Sigma products, such as Del Prado cheese and Yoplait yogurt. Sigma is a Mexican conglomerate with operations in eighteen countries. Sigma sells processed meats and cheese products and has international partnerships with Oscar Meyer (Europe), Sodima/Yoplait (France), Del Prado (Costa Rica), Zar (Costa Rica), Bar-S Foods Co. (United States), and Supremo (Mexico), among others (Sigma Alimentos 2019). Some cheese products are also exported to other countries in Central America, such as El Salvador and Nicaragua. These connections further highlight the way that this rural mountain community is part of the global economic market.

The Quakers settled in one area of the region known as Monteverde. They worked together with Ticos to build the community that exists today, which includes public and private schools as well as a community-centered nonprofit organization, the Monteverde Institute. The Monteverde Institute's mission statement was developed formally in 1986 and was a collaborative effort between Quakers and Ticos to promote sustainable tourism in the Monteverde Zone (Monteverde Institute n.d.). Ticos and Quakers worked together from the 1970s on to make sure that conservation was a top priority for the area, which now has numerous private reserves (Honey 2008). This contributed to the ecotourism that exists today, as well as the education tourism in the form of student groups and individuals that come to the region to study or participate in local research in both the natural and the social sciences.

PAST RESEARCH IN THE MONTEVERDE ZONE

Research efforts have been ongoing in the Monteverde Zone since the formalization of the local conservation areas in the 1970s (Honey 2008). What originally started as research to explore themes of conservation and biodiversity (Crump et al. 1992; Santana 1984; Snow 1977; Feinsinger 1976) grew to include research on tourism (Stocker 2013), ecotourism (Honey 2008; Aylward et al. 1996), gender roles and social reproduction (Ferguson 2011, 2010), sexual behavior (Romero-Daza and Freidus 2008), mental health (Cowherd 2012), child growth and development (Ruiz 2015), pregnancy practices (Cantor et al. 2013), and food insecurity (Himmelgreen et al. 2014, 2013, 2006; Ruiz et al. 2014). With the opening of the Monteverde Institute, efforts to develop and guide sustainable tourism through community-based programs have brought educational groups to the Monteverde Zone. These groups often engage in local environmental or social research, such as the fifteen-year partnership with the University of South Florida. This has involved student research on various health topics, which include nutrition (Banks et al. 2010; Cantor et al. 2008), reproductive health (Furhmann et al. 2006; D'Epiro et al. 2002), and water and sanitation (Van Zee et al. 2014; Baker et al. 2006), and have directly influenced programs and services offered within the community, including the development of a local farmer's market, a women's physical activity program, and a community garden. This book builds on research in the Monteverde Zone exploring links between the shift to a tourism economy and food insecurity (Himmelgreen et al. 2014, 2013, 2006). Himmelgreen and colleagues (2006) originally found that food insecurity was high in the Monteverde Zone within their sample and reached 73 percent in the study community that was most integrated into the tourism economy. This study examined the relationship between food insecurity and other variables and found that body mass index, not having a working stove, and not being a member of a food cooperative were all predictors of food insecurity. Additionally, researchers found that there was an inverse association between food insecurity and condiment consumption, highlighting concerns of dietary delocalization (i.e., the incorporation of nonlocal food items in the diet and diminishing autonomy of local food production [Pelto and Pelto 1983]) and food access among some segments of the population. This study prompted University of South Florida researchers to apply for a National Science Foundation grant, which they received, and allowed them to conduct more in-depth research on food insecurity in the region over a three-year period, from 2009 to 2011. Some results show that approximately half of study participants (51%) were food insecure in the thirty days prior to the interview (Himmelgreen et al. 2014). Further, in-depth interviews revealed five factors that contributed to food-related decision-making. This includes (1) food prices, (2) work patterns, (3) food access and availability, (4) social support systems, and (5) food preferences. These findings are particularly relevant to understanding how the recent political-economic shifts have affected local diets, as the increases in wage work and rising food prices influence the access and availability of certain food items. Further, with increased flow of cultural ideas as a result of globalization and interaction with tourists, the social structure and local food preferences may be shifting. Another researcher from the University of South Florida, Ernesto Ruiz (2014), explored the relationship between food insecurity and physical growth and development among children. His work found that there was an inverse relationship between these two variables, as children from food secure households in the sample tended to be shorter and had shorter leg lengths. Ruiz (2014) suggests dietary quality may be responsible for these findings. Ruiz noted that as children in food secure households are getting enough to eat in terms of quantity, these foods may be lacking in quality, as packaged and processed high caloric food items often are. On the other hand, children in food insecure households do not have the quantity they require but, as Ruiz indicated, may be getting the quality by consuming nutritious foods. In the work conducted by Himmelgreen and colleagues (2014, 2006), the majority of participants were women, which led to the development of my own preliminary research (Cantor et al. 2013). That study explored the links between tourism and maternal diet and found that women were concerned about maternal overweight/obesity and pregnancy practices were changing. Women described foods of the past as "healthier" and "from the land," whereas diets today were increasingly comprised of processed foods like pizza and fried chicken. Additionally, women indicated that sources of information about pregnancy practices were shifting from their families to the local clinic. Although women have access to modern medicine because of the local clinic, they have also lost cultural practices, such as *cuarentena*, a designated postpartum period with specific dietary and behavioral prescriptions and taboos traditionally observed to promote bonding between mothers and their offspring, and to mitigate the negative health consequences of adverse ecological stressors (e.g., cold weather, rain, etc.) (Alarcón and Nahuelcheo 2008; Piperata 2008; de la Torre and Rush 1987). Additionally, there were indications that this area was experiencing a nutrition transition. This book builds on the previous work conducted in the Monteverde Zone and contributes to a broader understanding of maternal health in the context of rapid global development. The emphasis on pregnancy health is important, as pregnancy is a critical developmental period for offspring and is a sensitive time for mothers as they experience decreased immune function to allow for the growth and development of their unborn children.

NOTE

1. Although the University of Costa Rica has visited the Monteverde Zone over the years to visually inspect specific sites and speak with the community about how to preserve artifacts, no large-scale excavations or surveys have taken place. Further, it is almost impossible to identify and catalogue material remains when taken out of context, which they are as soon as they are moved from the site where originally found. Local enthusiasts have been documenting findings and reviewing individuals' personal collections and discovered that some items were made with nonlocal materials, such as obsidian, indicating that trade and/or travel was occurring in this region.

Chapter 2

Tourism

As I put on my shoes I thanked the yoga instructor. I left the small yoga room and walked down the dusty and rocky unpaved road. I walked past the cow pastures, nodding to the cows as they stared at me with a far-off gaze. In less than ten minutes, I had arrived at the local nonprofit organization where I worked. I walked into the main office and got a strange look from one of the employees. She greeted me and then said, "You look like a tourist today." I looked down at my yoga clothes: Keen-brand, closed-toed hiking sandals, black yoga pants, a black nonprofit affiliate t-shirt, and a black name-brand sweater. I responded with, "Well I am a tourist!" The employee disagreed. However, another program assistant standing nearby chimed in, "Yeah, you are," as he smiled slyly. I had been working with the female employee for a few years and had known her since I started coming to the Monteverde Zone in 2008. This was my first time working with the male employee and we had only known each other for a few months. To some, I am merely a tourist. To others, my status has changed over the years, accounting for the surprise by my coworker that I looked like a tourist on this particular day. This example reflects the tensions that exist in defining the role of tourism and tourists in this community. While tourism certainly is not new to this region, locals still negotiate with what the continued presence of the tourism industry means for themselves and their community.

The Monteverde Zone is an established and well-known tourist destination due to its location in the Costa Rican cloud forest, an ecosystem which supports high levels of biodiversity. Although not everyone in the area is connected directly with the tourism industry, it permeates daily life indirectly through its relationship to infrastructural and economic development in the region as a whole. The social impacts are also notable, as identity politics come into play through everyday interactions, as the one described above.

Additionally, there is now an entire generation of locals that does not know the Monteverde Zone without tourism. As one of my participants noted, "Well, Monteverde has always depended on tourism. Always during my lifetime it has depended on tourism" (María, 18, 6 months pregnant[1]).

In 1974, the Monteverde Zone began to formally welcome tourists with the opening of the Monteverde Cloud Forest Reserve. Locals had noticed that more people were visiting region and began conservation efforts that resulted in the various reserves that still operate today. What began with 450 visitors now brings over 250,000 tourists to the region annually (Hamilton 2015; Himmelgreen et al. 2013; Honey 2008). Tourists come to enjoy the extreme biodiversity, as Costa Rica is home to approximately 4 percent of all the known plant and animal species in the world, but covers only 0.04 percent of the earth's surface (Monteverde Cloud Forest Reserve n.d.), which makes it a great place to see many species in a geographically small space. In general, tourists come to Costa Rica to see sloths, monkeys, and sea turtles. Nature enthusiasts who come to the region know that the Monteverde Zone is a corridor for various migratory birds, such as the resplendent quetzal and the three-wattled bellbird, and that plant diversity is extremely high.

HISTORICAL CONTEXT: CENTRAL AMERICA

The changes in the Monteverde Zone should be contextualized within the historical trajectory of tourism in Central America. Although tourism in Central America was not fully developed as an industry until the 1980s, the region's shared history set the stage for its ability to participate in the global market economy, which later fostered the tourism industry. The first common historical experience that united the region began in the sixteenth century when Central America entered into the world system via Spanish and British colonization (Robinson 1998).

Columbus first landed on the shores of Costa Rica in 1502, and his son described in his diary the "richness of the coast" of this new land, which would become "Costa Rica" (the rich coast) (Creedman 1991). Natural and labor resources were exploited during colonization as Spanish settlers and missionaries came to the area, which included agricultural production (e.g., cacao), raising of livestock (e.g., cows, mules, and horses), and forced indigenous labor (Palmer and Molina 2006). Although some indigenous labor was employed for small-scale farming, the spread out geographical nature of indigenous groups, as well as the thick tropical forests and mountainous terrain made it difficult to achieve levels of labor exploitation that occurred in other regions in Latin America (Waibel 1939). However, Spanish settlements used the encomienda system that was common throughout Latin America and required that the local indigenous population become evangelized and pay tribute to the crown with goods such as corn, beans, and honey (Molina and Palmer 2007). During the colonial period, goods from Costa Rica were exported throughout Latin America and included wood (e.g., cedar), food products (e.g., corn, honey, and beans), artisan products (e.g., hammocks, ceramics, and cotton threads), and livestock (e.g., cattle, pigs, and chickens) (Molina and Palmer 2007). What began as 55 Spanish families grew to 60,000 by the turn of the nineteenth century as the colonial period came to an end (Waibel 1939). In contrast, it is estimated that 120,000 indigenous peoples lived in Costa Rica in 1569 and by 1611 there were only 10,000 (Palmer and Molina 2006). Today, indigenous peoples account for about 2 percent of the total population (INEC 2011), representing eight indigenous groups. This colonial era population decline is attributed to war, disease, relocation, and exploitation (Palmer and Molina 2006). Eventually, power dynamics between the colonies and Spain shifted and rebellions and uprisings led to the formation of independent nation-states after the Mexican War of Independence in 1821 (Molina and Palmer 2007). This impacted Costa Rica since the newly formed nation-state of Mexico did not include Central America in its plans for nation building. After the Spanish were overthrown, Central America became independent and attempted to create what was called the Federal Republic of Central America, which included all the contemporary countries in this region, except for Panama (Molina and Palmer 2007).

Costa Rica adopted its own constitution as a sovereign nation in 1848 (Molina and Palmer 2007). The country then became an "agro-export" society like the rest of Central America during this time (Torres Rivas 1993, cited in Robinson 1998), which brought lucrative big businesses to the region through the production and exportation of commodity items such as coffee and bananas, as well as through participation in the garment industry. In Costa Rica, enterprises like America's United Fruit Company exploited resources as well as the local population through business practices that would not have lasted in the United States due to changing attitudes regarding labor rights around the turn of the twentieth century (Koeppel 2007). It was this endeavor that created the high demand for bananas in the United States, since banana companies started widespread campaigns to sell bananas on a large commercial scale. Bananas had previously been a luxury item since the technology did not exist to keep them fresh as they traveled from the Caribbean to the United States (Koeppel 2007). Banana barons invested in different technologies that would improve the market for bananas, such as building railroads throughout Central America, creating radio networks (to permit communication between plantations and cargo vessels), and inventing refrigeration technology for their fleets (Koeppel 2007). Growth of industry continued and agricultural exports remained the dominant source of financial capital until the 1970s, when the Central American economy began to transform as the region became increasingly integrated into the global market through new economic opportunities such as maquiladora production, tourism, nontraditional exports, and remittances (Robinson 1998). Following the historical trend in the area, the development of the tourism industry was made possible by transnational stakeholders, as funding was provided by the World Bank and other international organizations (e.g., USAID) (Honey 2008; O'Neill 2002). The financial restructuring of loans from these organizations in the 1980s was a major contributor to the Latin American debt crisis, emphasizing the way that power relationships have continually maintained the oppressor/subordinate relationship in this region (Adams et al. 2013).

Although the history of outside domination and exploitation in Central America continues today, Costa Rica followed a different trajectory than the other countries in the region. In contrast to political instability and poor social and living conditions resulting from conflict and war that occurred in other countries (e.g., Guatemala and Honduras), Costa Rica has remained a stable political body since it abolished its army (Molina and Palmer 2007). As a result of social reforms in the 1970s, which were ultimately backed financially by revenue from Costa Rica's participation in the global market economy, social services were developed, including access to clean water, socialized health care, and education, that reached most of its citizens (Muñoz and Scrimshaw 1995). Additionally, without an army, Costa Rica was able to draw on resources that would have been otherwise used for national defense. Health and social well-being improved dramatically during the 1970s, and within a few decades, key health indicators were improved. For example, infant mortality dropped from 61.1/1,000 in 1970 to 19.1/1,000 in 1990 (Muñoz and Valverde 1995), to 7.8/1,000 in 2017 (PAHO 2017). These changes also resulted in increased access to health care throughout most of the country (Muñoz and Scrimshaw 1995). Good social indicators helped to lure tourists to the region. In 1980, the tourism industry generated $81 million in revenue and by 1989 it was a $201 million industry, with North Americans and Europeans accounting for more than half of this (Coffey 1993). Today, the estimated value of the tourism industry in Costa Rica is approaching $4 billion (ICT 2017). The Costa Rican government quickly saw the economic potential of tourism, and in 1985 the Tourism Investment Incentives Law was developed, which provided economic benefits and incentives to businesses that catered exclusively to tourists. This includes hotels, tourist-oriented air and water transport companies, car rental agencies, and travel agencies (Coffey 1993). These incentives attracted attention from multinational companies in the 1980s and 1990s, which helped to boost tourism with economic investment in infrastructure and advertisements (Ferguson 2010). Today, tourism directly employs 5.1 percent of the labor force and contributes to 12.5 percent of employment overall (World Travel & Tourism Council 2018) and accounts for 6.7 percent of the gross domestic product (ICT 2017).

Ecotourism has become a popular form of tourism in Costa Rica due to the incredible biodiversity in the country. Honey (2008) distinguishes ecotourism from other types of tourism (e.g., nature tourism), as "it goes further, in striving to respect and benefit protected areas as well as the people living around or on these lands" (Loc 77). In addition to ecotourism, various other forms of tourism have also become popular. This includes adventure tourism (i.e., focused on adventure recreation) (Weber 2001), medical tourism (Warf 2010) (i.e., "a combination of leisure travel and invasive biomedical procedures, in which poorer countries offer visitors from wealthier countries an appealing package of state-of-the-art clinical services, hospitable locals, and exotic sightseeing" [Ackerman 2010, 404]), sex tourism (Frohlick 2016; Rivers-Moore 2016) (i.e., "travel to specific sites with the intent to engage in sexual relations with local residents" [Romero-Daza and Freidus 2008, 1]), and educational tourism (i.e., tourism with the purpose of education and learning) (Myers et al. 2005; Ritchie et al. 2003).

Ecotourism has boomed in Costa Rica due to both its location in the tropics and conservation efforts in the 1970s and 1980s, which expanded protected land (Monteverde Cloud Forest n.d.; Horton 2009). Today, protected land makes up more than a quarter of the total land in Costa Rica (CCSA 2018). This policy change reflected global concern at the time about the decimation of tropical forests in Latin America due to illegal mining, logging, ranching, oil drilling, and human settlement; it also contributed to the boom in ecotourism (Honey 2008). Additionally, Oscar Arias, the former president of Costa Rica, won the Nobel Peace Prize in 1987 for his efforts to promote peace in Central America. Arias's efforts put Costa Rica in the global spotlight as a peaceful mecca in the war-torn Latin America (Honey 2008).[2]

Costa Rica has been described as "a global destination for pleasure tourism associated with nature, purity, health-enhancement, and the bodily" (Frohlick 2013, 134). Ironically, the local impacts of tourism sometimes contradict this view and are overlooked by foreign visitors (Zúniga 2009). "Critics [of ecotourism] contend, however, that, as Costa Rica's latest transnational activity, ecotourism perpetuates historical patterns of inequality, social exclusion, and environmental degradation associated with past patterns of dependent, agro-export led growth in Central America" (Horton 2009, 94). Horton (2009) argues that ecotourism is a political process, involving power struggles (e.g., access to land, natural resources, economic benefits, representations of the environment, and quality of life). This is exemplified by the wealth gap between foreign tourists and locals. Sixty-eight percent of North American and European tourists have a college degree and 36 percent have an average income of over $100,000 (*Tico Times* survey cited in Horton 2009), while the average income for a Costa Rican household is approximately $16,863.20 annually (ENAHO 2019). Further, a study about ecotourism in the Osa Peninsula, a popular tourist destination in southern Costa Rica, found "unequal distributional impacts and practices and beliefs of competition, individualism, material accumulation, consumption, and commodification. Such processes may disempower local peoples, fragmenting communities, limiting collective action, and restraining imaginings of qualitatively different forms of development" (Horton 2009, 100). Still, there are some that argue that ecotourism benefits local livelihood, and in some cases alleviates poverty (Hunt et al. 2015). In the Quaker settlement of Monteverde, which has a history of community activism and a "participatory, town-meeting style of governance" (Honey 2008, 191), tourism has brought changes in wealth differences, among other things. Nat Scrimshaw, a previous director of the Monteverde Institute, explains, "In the past, there was a lot of moral force that acted to shape whether something happened or somebody did something. And that is simply no longer true, now there's not time, and it's too diverse. And that has been pulling at the texture of the traditional town meeting that used to run everything" (Honey 2008, 191). Ferguson (2011) notes that increased tourism in the Monteverde Zone has also led to restructuring of traditional power dynamics, such as those found in gender, class, ethnicity, and nationality relations. In addition, income inequality in Costa Rica has risen since the 1980s due to shifts in work patterns (Gindling and Trejos 2005; ENAHO 2018). Increased inequality results in differential access to nutritional resources (Drewnowski 2009; Otero et al. 2015; Gustafson et al. 2016), and as individuals favor economic endeavors over traditional lifestyles, access to, availability of, and desire for specific food resources changes.

However, in the Monteverde Zone, many locals view ecotourism, and tourism in general, as a positive force in the community. As a direct result of ecotourism, private conservation areas have been developed to promote sustainability and research (Honey 2008; Aylward et al. 1995). Additionally, locals view tourism as an important source of income, as well as an opportunity for cross-cultural learning (Himmelgreen et al. 2014, 2006). The latter phenomenon often occurs during interactions with tourists through activities such as local homestay programs, where tourists live with locals for a period of time. In the past, locals have indicated that they have learned about healthy eating habits, such as consuming green salads (Himmelgreen et al. 2014), as well as other cultures or religions, such as Judaism, which do not have a strong presence in the region. While overall, locals have a positive perception of tourism in the Monteverde Zone, they do indicate that there are some negative aspects, such as the increase in prices of goods and services and the dependency on tourism, which has led some to abandon agriculture in favor of increased participation in the market economy through tourism activities (Himmelgreen et al. 2014).

The shift from agricultural subsistence and dairy farming to a mixed economy that relies heavily on tourism brought changes to the zone, such as the establishment of local and international businesses that have increased local access to various goods and services, such as chain supermarkets. However, contemporaneous dietary delocalization, food insecurity, and the rise in chronic noncommunicable diseases have also been noted (Cantor et al. 2013; Himmelgreen et al. 2014, 2013, 2006). There is also evidence that the Monteverde Zone, like other parts of the world, is experiencing a nutrition transition, which is linked with rapid development (Cantor et al. 2013). Shifting political economy and the subsequent nutrition transition have changed the social and cultural values surrounding specific food items, and the neoliberal agenda and commodification of food items have influenced food availability, access, and utilization (Asfaw 2008; Hawkes 2008), leading to food insecurity for some households.

FOOD INSECURITY

Food security is defined "as existing when all people at all times have access to sufficient, safe, nutritious food to maintain a healthy and active life. Commonly, the concept of food security is defined as including both physical and economic access to food that meets people's dietary needs as well as their food preferences" (WHO 2016a). In Latin America, 9.8 percent of the population suffers from severe food insecurity (WHO 2018). Vulnerability to food insecurity has been described as the relationship between risk and the ability/capability to cope (Martinez et al. 2009), which has implications for shifting access to resources as a result of increasing socioeconomic stratification linked with tourism. Today, globalization and transnational processes have created a situation that moves beyond the lack of food availability. It has been noted that in Latin America food insecurity is due to issues of access and utilization, rather than availability (Rose 2008). This is reflected in the Monteverde Zone. While residents once fully relied on subsistence agriculture, today many households that have transitioned to rely on a tourism economy still grow produce and use milk from their dairy cattle to make cheese and yogurt. However, studies show that food insecurity is high in some areas (Himmelgreen et al. 2006). Intrahousehold dynamics can also influence the effects of food insecurity, as women have been noted to buffer their children from unhealthy diets in the context of food insecurity, compromising their own health in the process (Schmeer et al. 2014; McIntyre et al. 2003) and women suffer from higher rates of severe food insecurity than men in Latin America (WHO 2018). In addition, past and present economic disadvantages (i.e., poverty) are associated with food insecurity (WHO 2018; Sarlio-Lähteenkorva and Lahelma 2001; Maxwell 1998), and as more individuals enter the wage labor force, social stratification increases (Leatherman and Goodman 2005). In line with aspects of the nutrition transition, processed, packaged nonlocal food items that are part of the global food industrial complex are often cheaper, or become cheaper, than locally grown fruits and vegetables (Hawkes 2008; Pratt 2007; Cantor et al. 2018). The increase in supermarkets throughout Latin America also contributes to this, providing a source of cheap energy-dense, low-nutrient foods (Asfaw 2008; Reardon et al. 2003).

Increased reliance on tourism as a source of economic capital can be problematic when there is seasonality in the industry. In the Monteverde Zone, Himmelgreen and colleagues (2006) found that food insecurity was high and may be related to the flux in the tourist season. Since some households relied on tourism for cash wages, during the low tourism season work may be scarcer, bringing in less income to spend on food. The shift to a tourism-dominant economy has decreased the reliance on agriculture in the region and increased a reliance on store-bought food items. The high prices of store-bought items are attributed to dietary delocalization, with many items coming from outside of the zone, and the desire to benefit economically from tourism. However, as Himmelgreen and colleagues' (2006) participants indicated, the prices remain high, even in the low season. As one of their participants noted, "When tourism decreases so do the jobs. . . . Then the situation turns difficult. I don't have enough money to buy my kids and myself what I want. One could buy the same foods but in smaller amounts" (308). The lack of diversity in livelihood strategies is also associated with food insecurity since there is less flexibility in the ability to cope with different stressors (Hanazaki et al. 2013). The high prices and reliability on seasonality of work influence the capability of households to purchase some foods, ultimately influencing consumption patterns, diet quality, and energy balance.

FOOD INSECURITY AND PREGNANCY

Although food insecurity poses a health risk to the entire population, pregnant women can be considered particularly vulnerable to the negative consequences. Prenatal energy requirements are different than the general population and include an increased consumption of many micronutrients, such as iron and vitamin B (ACOG 2018), as well as a moderate increase in macronutrients and overall calories (approximately 300 kilocalories daily) (APA 2019). Research shows that among food insecure households women might experience a reduction in micronutrient intake (Park and Eicher-Miller 2014; Fischer et al. 2006; McIntyre et al. 2003; Tarasuk and Beaton 1999; Rose and Oliveira 1997), increase in overweight and obesity (Papan and

Clow 2015; Franklin et al. 2012; Adams et al. 2003; Olson 1999), and difficulty in returning to their pregravid (i.e., prepregnancy) weight (Laraia et al. 2015; Olson and Strawderman 2008). However, causality among these relationships is often unclear (Ives and Cullen 2011). This is the case with obesity, as Olson and Strawderman (2008) have identified this as a factor that leads to food insecurity, as opposed to the other way around.

Among pregnant women, there can be an increase in pregravid overweight and obesity, gestational diabetes (Laraia et al. 2010), birth defects (Carmichael et al. 2007), and poor pregnancy outcomes associated with stress that often accompanies food insecurity (Dolatian et al. 2018; Borders et al. 2007; Laraia et al. 2006;Whitaker et al. 2006). Maternal overweight and obesity, gestational diabetes, birth defects, and stress are linked with inadequate dietary quality (i.e., intake of micro and macronutrients) (Laraia et al. 2010; Carmichael et al. 2007). Additionally, psychosocial stress related to coping with unstable food conditions can cause depression, anxiety, and general stress during the prenatal and postnatal period (Power et al. 2017; Laraia et al. 2015, 2006; Hromi-Fiedler et al. 2011). The consequences of food insecurity can cause proximal health impacts on the mother and her child, such as poor birth outcomes (Dolatian et al. 2018). Food insecurity can also have distal effects on health, such as poor-quality maternal-child interactions (Frith et al. 2012), insults to developmental pathways associated with stress response and metabolic functioning (Glover 2014; Lau et al. 2011), and impacts on offspring diet and nutrition (Gross et al. 2018).

MATERNAL DIET

Dietary delocalization, wage labor, and the cross-cultural exchange of ideas regarding food and consumption also influence maternal diet. High socioeconomic status has been linked with specific chronic conditions, such as overweight/obesity, although some research has found that transitional communities, which are undergoing modernization and often have lower socioeconomic status also exhibit higher rates of chronic noncommunicable diseases as diet and lifestyles change rapidly with increased access to cash and dietary delocalization (Arps 2011; Bosu 2015; Jaacks et al. 2017). The reliance on cash, high prices of food, and limited livelihood strategies contribute to changes in maternal diet in areas experiencing a nutrition transition. Hawkes (2008) discusses the roles of supermarkets in shaping individual and group dietary patterns and concludes that supermarkets encourage consumers to eat more, since this will be profitable for business. Asfaw (2008) found that in Guatemala the presence of supermarkets did increase consumption of processed foods. Women in Central America are responsible for the domestic sphere, including most food preparation. Therefore, increased access to supermarkets directly affects women's dietary choices, influencing energy balance, diet quality, and consumption patterns. This is exacerbated by the increased economic opportunities for women, which bring them into the public sphere where they consume meals of convenience that fit with their new work schedules. In the Monteverde Zone, two grocery stores, both of which are subsidiaries of the large conglomerates, Gessa and MegaSuper, now provide locals with access to commodity food items, including a plethora of packaged, energy-dense foods that are produced, distributed, and sold by large transnational corporations. In a preliminary study in the Monteverde Zone, my colleagues and I (Cantor et al. 2013) found that mothers of young children (younger than ten years old) reported craving foods such as French fries, pizza, and store-bought desserts during pregnancy. In contrast, mothers with older children (older than twenty years old) reported craving and consuming foods such as fruits, fish, and vegetables. The mothers with older children explained that when they were pregnant they did not have access to supermarkets or many restaurants, and everything they ate came from the land. Mothers with both younger and older children also discussed weight gain as a problem for mothers today. In this case, consumption patterns were altered by the nutrition transition via tourism development and may have had an impact on desire for specific foods, dietary quality, and energy balance, resulting in increased rates of overweight and obesity. Himmelgreen and colleagues (2014, 2013, 2006) also noted high rates of overweight and obesity among women in their studies, which is consistent with other literature from Latin America that shows disproportionately higher rates of overweight and obesity among women than men (Popkin and Reardon 2018; Uauy and Monteiro 2004; Kain et al. 2003; Filozof et al. 2001; Martorell et al. 1998). I argue that since pregnancy is a unique experience within the life course for women, rooted in specific cultural contexts and ideologies, the nutrition transition may not adequately predict the ways that pregnancy health will be affected. Research should focus on the ways that the nutrition transition impacts pregnancy health within specific cultural contexts, as this book does.

NOTES

1. Participants are always referred to using pseudonyms and their age. For pregnant women, there is always a lot of discussion about how many months pregnant they are (i.e., *cuánto tiene*?) and so this information is included as well.
2. While Oscar Arias has been lauded for his efforts at peacekeeping in Central America, he has recently been accused of sexual assault, which has made him a contentious political figure.

Chapter 3

The Nutrition Transition

The wood fire crackled and popped as smoke billowed from the large aluminum olla (cooking pot). The sweet smell of condensed milk filled the air and was laden with hints of cinnamon. I barely fit with Mariella and her seven-year-old daughter as we crammed into the small storage shack that housed the *cocina de leña*, or wood stove, in the backyard. I watched as Mariella moved the flaming logs around with a stick, constantly readjusting to make sure the olla was getting just the right amount of heat. Mariella explained to me that the traditional Costa Rican dish, *arroz con leche* (rice pudding), always tasted better when cooked on the *cocina de leña*, and that is why she chose not to use the modern gas stove in the kitchen. I arrived late and she already had the rice cooking with cinnamon sticks and was periodically adding milk. Mariella had a fixed eye on the steaming dish, stirring it every few minutes so that it wouldn't burn. I watched her slowly add a can of Nestle sweetened condensed milk as we chatted, then another. I wondered how many cans she added so far. I also wondered what she thought about the nutritional value of this dish. This was a specialty after all, not something that was consumed every day, but still, I couldn't help but wonder what the common attitudes were concerning nutrition. These are the same thoughts I had in the clinic when the sugary snack was served to the pregnant women and their partners. Although some foods like *arroz con leche* were only meant for special and celebratory occasions, the Ticos I knew in the Monteverde Zone were always finding things to celebrate. If there was nothing to celebrate, there was always the *hora de café*, or coffee hour, which was observed daily at some time in the afternoon and included coffee or tea and a snack (e.g., *prestiños* [fried dough] with honey or *arepas* [pancakes]). The *arroz con leche* was finished just in time for the *hora de café*. While it cooled, Mariella prepared *café chorreado*. Mariella dumped heaping spoonful after spoonful of ground coffee into the reusable cloth filter, which fit snugly in the metal stand. As she poured the boiling water through the filter she stirred the coffee grounds periodically. The large metal cup that caught the coffee was steaming and filled the air with the strong aroma of fresh brew. Mariella offered me sugar and powdered milk as she absentmindedly added two overflowing spoons of sugar into her cup. I wondered why she chose powdered milk over fresh milk, this area was known for their dairy farms after all. It's possible that this processed alternative was cheaper and more accessible to her. The *arroz con leche* was ready. As we ate, Mariella continuously asked me if I wanted more, even though my bowl was full. I ate slowly, as the dish was very sweet. I also wondered how much sugar she added, or if the sweetness I tasted was from the condensed milk.

Although this example speaks to the cultural constitution of foods, it does not necessarily reflect ideas about the nutritional value of foods, or how culturally situated ideas about nutrition inform actual dietary practices and influence health. I found this to be lacking from everyday conversation and narrative regarding food in the Monteverde Zone, although this is a crucial piece of information when it comes to understanding the relationship between food-related decision-making and nutritional changes brought on by the tourism-driven nutrition transition. In this example, it's clear that biology and culture are intertwined in a delicate dance choreographed by political-economic forces. While Mariella prepared a local and traditional dish, some of the ingredients she used have been delocalized, such as the Nestle sweetened condensed milk and the powdered milk she used instead of local cow's milk. This has nutritional implications, for example, sweetened condensed milk contains added refined sugars. This example also illustrates how globalized practices, such as participation in the industrial food system, impact local practices, such as food preparation. While the nutrition transition is directly responsible for macro-level shifts in how we, as a global society, think about and consume food, the idea that humans are active agents of these changes is often left out of the narrative. Further, the nutrition transition framework doesn't account for the localized ways that biology and culture interact to affect health. The CBCA in anthropology brings together the various themes noted here, namely, the way that political-economic forces interact with biology and culture. This framework is useful for drawing connections between global processes and local, lived realities and the dialectical between the two. However, the role of human agency in shaping these environments is also absent from studies that employ the CBCA.

During my first visit to the Monteverde Zone in 2008 I noticed that while this rural community was deeply entrenched in global practices, such as the increasing presence of "fast foods" like pizza, hamburgers, and French fries, many locals did not eat out. During the month that I participated in a homestay experience with a local family there was only one occasion on which the family went out to eat. For the last meal with my *madre tica* (Costa Rican "mom") we went to lunch at a local hotel where she had familial ties. We ate salad with hearts of palm and *casados*, a traditional Costa Rican dish comprised of rice, beans, and a protein. In this example, as well as the one above, individuals were active agents in negotiating with changes to the food environment in the region (brought on by the global nutrition transition), while drawing on their own cultural identity to make decisions about how to prepare food, where to eat, and what to eat. This book contributes to an understanding of the relationship between the global age in which we live and everyday experiences by bringing human agency into the broader dialogue about the local impacts of the worldwide nutrition transition. In addition, the application and operationalization of practice theory in the context of the CBCA is a unique contribution to the field of medical anthropology and biocultural studies on health.

NUTRITION TRANSITION

The nutrition transition is marked by the shift to a more "Western" diet and lifestyle, which includes increased consumption of cooking oils, animal-source foods, caloric sweeteners, and packaged and processed foods, accompanied by decreased physical activity (Popkin et al. 2012; Bermudez and Tucker 2003; Drewnowski and Popkin 1997). First coined by Popkin in the early 1990s (Popkin 1994; Popkin et al. 1993), "nutrition transition" seemed to be an appropriate way to explain the shifting epidemiological profile worldwide. The shift from infectious disease to chronic noncommunicable disease was part of what Omran (1971) originally described as the epidemiologic transition. Popkin (2002) contextualized these health changes in the context of nutrition and detailed various stages of the nutrition transition, which include (1) collecting food, (2) famine, (3) receding famine, (4) nutrition-related noncommunicable disease, and (5) behavioral change (Dufour and Bender 2013). This model has been widely applied since the 1990s, mostly focusing on stage four, and has been used to explain contemporary health trends (e.g., the rise in overweight and obesity) (Popkin and Reardon 2018; Popkin et al. 2012; Astrup et al. 2008; Hawkes 2006; Schmidhuber and Shetty 2005; Popkin 2002), explore differences between high-income and low/middle-income countries (Popkin 1994), explain patterns of diet-associated nutritional change within a regional and global context (Popkin 2004; Rivera et al. 2004; Albala et al. 2001; Popkin et al. 1993), and to connect global economic processes with local public health initiatives (Thow 2009; Thow and Hawkes 2009; Hawkes and Thow 2008; Rayner et al. 2006).

Stage four is characterized by the high consumption of fats (e.g., cooking oils), cholesterol, sugars, refined carbohydrates, and a decreased intake of fiber and polyunsaturated fats. This has been linked with the "reliance upon processed foods, increased away-from-home food intake, and increased use of edible oils and sugar-sweetened beverages" (Popkin et al. 2012, 3). In stage four, the prevalence of obesity rises, leading to an increase in diet-related chronic noncommunicable disease. The fifth stage involves changes in diet to resemble those of stage one. "This stage is unique in that it involves conscious purposeful changes in nutrition and physical activity" (Dufour and Bender 2013).

Nutrition Transition and Health

The global health trend previously described (i.e., the shift to diet-related chronic noncommunicable disease) is described as increased rates of cardiovascular disease, type 2 diabetes, metabolic syndrome, overweight, and obesity, which have been recorded over the last twenty to thirty years, during the period of the rapid shift to the global market economy (Popkin et al. 2012; Amuna and Zotor 2008). Although there is not one pathway through which these chronic noncommunicable diseases manifest, there are a variety of mechanisms through which the nutrition transition affects disease risk. Diet is inextricably linked with nutrition, as consumption patterns influence an individual's or group's nutritional status (i.e., intake of micro and macronutrients and kilocalories). Nutrition is an important indicator of overall health, and during pregnancy, nutrition plays an important role in growth and development of offspring and the maintenance of maternal health. This book focuses on food insecurity and characteristics of maternal diet (i.e., consumption patterns) in relation to the nutrition transition (i.e., consumption of animal-source foods, sugars and caloric sweeteners, and packaged and processed foods) and participation in the tourism economy in order to explore the potential links between diet, nutrition, and health during the prenatal period.

Costa Rica experienced a nutrition and epidemiological transition concomitantly with the rise in tourism, which has been attributed to large-scale health reforms in the 1970s (Morgan 1990). There was a rapid decline in morbidity and mortality throughout the 1970s, which had a particularly strong impact on child mortality. Additionally, child malnutrition decreased dramatically during this time and was followed by an increase in population level chronic noncommunicable disease from the late 1980s to the present (del Rocío Sáenz et al. 2011; Araya and Padilla 2004). Today, 30 percent of mortality is due to cardiovascular disease, followed by cancer, and other chronic noncommunicable diseases (WHO 2011). Morbidity and mortality rates became more similar to industrialized countries than other countries in Central America, and today, Costa Rica is considered an upper middle-income country, with many social indicators on par with high-income countries, such as a 97.8 percent literacy rate and life expectancy of 77.7 percent for males and 82.4 percent for females (PAHO 2015, 2019). Further, overweight and obesity affects 25.7 percent of the population (WHO 2018) and has increased almost twofold among women since the 1980s (Agüero 2009). The increase in chronic non-communicable disease can be attributed to a variety of factors that are in line with characteristics of the nutrition transition, such as sedentary behaviors, body mass index (i.e., overweight and obesity), low fiber intake (between 11 and 25 grams total), increased fat consumption (Araya and Padilla 2004), and increased consumption of refined carbohydrates (Quesada and Gómez 2018; Fisberg et al. 2018; Kovalskys et al. 2018).

Tourism

Trends are similar throughout Central America. Research from the anthropological and public health literature on tourism in Central America suggests that increased participation in wage labor (due to tourism) and subsequent increased access to cash, as well as dietary delocalization and the cross-cultural exchange of knowledge, have worked in concert to facilitate the nutrition transition in this region. Increased participation in the tourism economy occurs as local communities grow to meet the demands of tourists (Himmelgreen et al. 2014, 2006; Leatherman et al. 2010, 2005; Wilson 2008; Key 2002). This not only means that individuals are working outside of the home more often but also that more women are entering into the workforce, particularly in areas experiencing urbanization (Cowherd 2012; Wilson 2008; Gentry 2007; Schmidhuber and Shetty 2005; Lundgren 1993). With women finding more opportunities outside of the domestic sphere, there is less time for intensive food preparations, opening the door for reliance on more convenient, store-bought food items. This includes precooked foods (e.g., frozen foods) or convenient snack items consumed outside of the home (Schmidhuber and Shetty 2005). Anthropologists working in the Yucatan found that the development of the tourism industry created a mixed economy of wage work and traditional milpa agriculture, which resulted in an increased reliance on urban areas for income generation and a decreased dependence on home gardens and traditional forms of subsistence (Leatherman et al. 2010). Increased access to cash also increases households' and individuals' ability to purchase food items outside of the home, as income is a major driver of food access, availability, and food demand (Uauy and Monteiro 2004). Consumption of animal products (e.g., meats and dairy products) also increases while consumption of complex carbohydrates as well as some grains, legumes, and other sources of fiber decreases (Uauy and Monteiro 2004). As restaurants and supermarkets open, local communities begin to have access to these foods, many of which are popular for tourists (Cantor et al. 2013; Asfaw 2008; Hawkes 2008; Schmidhuber and Shetty 2005; Reardon et al. 2003). Additionally, this is linked with the global industrial food complex, which has catered to, and at the same time has facilitated, the increased consumption of animal products (Hawkes 2008; Schmidhuber and Shetty 2005) and is associated with dietary delocalization.

In the Monteverde Zone, the reliance on agricultural products and home gardens has decreased and residents buy most of what they consume at the supermarket (Himmelgreen et al. 2006). Locals continue to complain about the high prices at the grocery store and the seasonality of food, and the tourism industry is problematic because prices remain high even when the tourism season is low and when there is typically less work available (Himmelgreen et al. 2006). In general, dietary delocalization occurs through infrastructure development and the appearance and continued presence of restaurants, supermarkets, bars, a wide range of accommodations (from hotels to hostels), souvenir shops, and tourist services (i.e., transportation, tours, etc.) (Asfaw 2008; Hawkes 2008; Reardon et al. 2003). These processes are ultimately linked with macro-level economic interests as participation in the global market economy increases, as is the case with tourism. Investment in the development of these establishments comes from local, national, and international outlets, the allocation of which affects local power structures and community dynamics. Desire for investments comes from a number of sources, which includes government incentives as well as macro-level trade liberalization. For example, the General Agreement on Trade in Services, implemented by the World Trade Organization, supports investment in the tourism industry "through easing restrictions relating to the flow of people, and thus facilitating consumption abroad and access to tourist destinations. The implications of this for food relate to the introduction of nontraditional foods to cater for tourists, as well as changes to agriculture as a result of a shift to a service economy" (Thow 2009, 2154).

Dietary delocalization is so pronounced in some regions that anthropologists working in the Yucatan have coined the term "coca-colonization" to refer to the commodification of food items and the high consumption of sugared beverages, such as Coca-Cola (Leatherman and Goodman 2005). This trend has been noted elsewhere in Central America, and in South America, the Caribbean, and Asia (Nagata et al. 2011). This concept was applied to dietary changes among the Tz'utujil Maya of Guatemala, as researchers found that inclusion of Coca-Cola in the diet has shaped health beliefs, religion, culture, and the environment (Nagata et al. 2011). For example, Coca-Cola was hybridized into the diet and came to be used for medicinal remedies (in combination with other herbs), included in festival cooking recipes, and was even offered with specific prayers (Nagata et al. 2011). In Costa Rica, researchers found that the consumption of commercially available fruit drinks and soda is associated with a higher body mass index and waist-to-hip ratio than consumption of traditional *frescos* (a beverage made of fresh fruit and water) (Rhee et al. 2012). Their findings were based on data from a ten-year study on heart disease and diet among Costa Rican adults, which enrolled 2,274 patients, 27 percent of whom were women. Although the authors did not directly link these findings with tourism, access and availability of store-bought fruit drinks, sodas, and a variety of cooking oils, even in rural areas, is inextricably linked with globalization.

Cross-cultural Examples

The cross-cultural transmission of ideas about nutrition and dietary habits also contributes to the nutrition transition. However, the literature on Central America is limited. In a study on the Garifuna of Roatan, researchers conclude that the commodification of culture through tourism leads to a loss of culture (Kirtsoglou and Theodossopoulos 2004). Participants argue that since they do not have control over this commodification, cross-cultural exchanges lead to an appropriation of their cultural traditions. In the classic case from the Yucatan already mentioned, anthropologists discuss food commodification and state that, "symbols of prestige become more Western" (Leatherman and Goodman 2005, 834) as tourism in the region ensues. Cross-culturally, tourism, particularly in more rural areas, has been associated with subsequent diet and lifestyle shifts characteristic of stage four of the nutrition transition (Himmelgreen et al. 2014, 2013, 2006; Leatherman et al. 2010; Cantor et al. 2013; Cantor et al. 2018; Dancause et al. 2012; Leatherman and Goodman 2005; Tessier and Gerber 2005; Daltabuit and Leatherman 1998). In the Mediterranean, researchers found that British colonization, migration, and tourism fostered a cultural interaction that ultimately impacted dietary habits on Malta (Tessier and Gerber 2005). However, in Sardinia this was less pronounced. Tourism began later, occurred on a smaller scale, and the percentage of foreign tourists was also low (21.4%) and dominated by other Mediterranean visitors (French and Spanish), as opposed to Anglo-Saxons, which resulted in local dietary habits remaining more stable. In the South Pacific, a similar trend has also been noted (Dancause et al. 2011; Bolabola 1981). Dietary data from the archipelago of Vanuatu in the South Pacific show increased consumption of animal proteins (i.e., meat and fish) and refined carbohydrates (i.e., bread, crackers, and instant noodles) that are associated with tourism-related economic development, urbanization, and urban migration, which accounts for the rapid increase in chronic disease (e.g., overweight, obesity, and hypertension) since the 1980s (Dancause et al. 2011). In contrast, Wilk (1999) argues that in Belize, tastes and food preferences are becoming more localized in an increasingly transnational world because of their value as cultural capital, giving locals power in the context of shifting power dynamics as a result of transitioning political economy.

The Monteverde Zone

Research conducted in the Monteverde Zone between 2003 and 2004 shows that dietary trends are associated with a nutrition transition. Himmelgreen and colleagues (2013) found that overweight and obesity among caretakers (all women) in 148 households was high, and child anthropometry indicated that 5 percent were underweight, 12 percent were overweight, and 10 percent were obese. Further, 10 percent of children were growth stunted, although there were no statistically significant differences by gender, as is reported in other studies (Martorell and Zongrone 2012). Logistic regression models predicted 81.5 percent of the food insecurity, and predictors were limited availability of condiments, caregiver's body mass index, not owning a microwave, not owning a working stove, and not being a member of a food cooperative. These variables are in line with characteristics of the nutrition transition (e.g., increased consumption of energy-dense, packaged foods) and the impacts of globalization (e.g., differential use of technology and decreased reliance on local food systems). Differences in child height were statistically significant between those in food secure households compared with those in food insecure households, , whereas those in food secure households were taller (Himmelgreen et al. 2013). However, only 49 percent of households participated in tourism, indicating that the effects of the nutrition transition reach beyond the direct link with tourism. Another study showed similar trends, most notably that caregiver body mass index (all women) was high and that food insecurity may be linked with the flux in the tourist season (Himmelgreen et al. 2006).

Preliminary research conducted with pregnant and nursing women in 2009 found that maternal diet in the Monteverde Zone has shifted to include foods characteristic of the nutrition transition, such as store-bought fried chicken, pizza, and French fries (Cantor et al. 2013). Additionally, women noted that weight gain during and after pregnancy was an emerging concern in this community, linking nutritional intake with health outcomes (Cantor et al. 2013). By documenting changes related to food access and availability in the Monteverde Zone, as well as exploring women's contemporary pregnancy experiences, this book addresses the paucity in the nutrition transition literature on pregnancy health.

Critiques of the Nutrition Transition

The nutrition transition framework has been critiqued for being essentialist in its application within local settings (Piperata et al. 2011; Dodd 2011; Barrett et al. 1998). Although it has been documented globally and is associated with poor health outcomes (e.g., overweight/obesity, type 2 diabetes, and metabolic syndrome) (Webber et al. 2012; Popkin et al. 2012; Hawkes et al. 2004; Popkin 2004; Rivera et al. 2004; Uauy and Monteiro 2001), the concept of the nutrition transition has its share of critics who recognize the diversity in human populations, a fact which does not lend itself to simplistic cause-and-effect relationships (Dufour and Bender 2013; Abu-Saad et al. 2012; Dodd 2011; Piperata et al. 2011). An in-depth consideration of the ways that subpopulations are affected by the nutrition transition is needed in order to account for human biological, social, and cultural variation, as the impacts of these changes are not uniform across populations. Dodd (2011) explores the political ecology of the nutrition transition in Central America, emphasizing the point that changes in nutritional intake are part of dynamic processes that "cannot be reduced to simplified models" (119). Additionally, Dodd (2011) calls for a more nuanced understanding of how these processes play out at both the individual and household levels. To address these concerns, Dodd uses two case studies from Central America to construct a framework called the nutrient-deficient ecology model, which is meant to "improve our comprehension of cases where individuals and households are unable to access a sustained and appropriate balance of macronutrients and micronutrients necessary to achieve an adequate level of health" (130). Focusing on the Ribeirinhos, a mixed indigenous ethnic population in the Amazon, anthropologists explored the relationship between economic shifts and nutritional changes, finding that increased participation in the cash economy through various avenues (i.e., the Bolsa Familia program, selling the açaí fruit for industrial processing, and government pensions) influenced food sources and consumption, as locals began to rely on purchased foods and there was a reduction in fishing and hunting (Piperata et al. 2011). Although changes fit within the model of the nutrition transition, specific aspects of change did not, such as a decrease in energy intake. The researchers conclude that the traditional conceptualization of the nutrition transition may not apply in all settings, such as in rural and marginalized areas where their research was conducted. Similarly, Abu-Saad and colleagues (2012) found inconsistencies with applying the nutrition transition model among pregnant Bedouin Arabs in Israel, as overlapping nutrition transition stages may have accounted for the high rates of prepregnancy overweight and obesity (42%) coupled with inadequate macronutrient and micronutrient intakes. Dufour and Bender (2012) also critique the widespread application of the nutritional transition framework and "argue that the model ignores the significant variation within and between human populations in the past as well as the present, and in doing so limits our understanding of the very phases and transitions the model proposes to represent" (372). Even Popkin and his colleagues (2012) have acknowledged the shortcomings of the framework and a need for new directions, calling for an expanded model that includes the "dynamics of change, rather than simplistic cross-sectional perspectives" (4). And although Popkin and colleagues (2012) recognize that the overabundance of current research focused on women of childbearing age and preschoolers may be a limitation with the framework, to date, there has been little research conducted on the impacts of diet and lifestyle changes on pregnancy health and outcomes (Abu-Saad et al. 2012), or the application of life history theory to understanding adverse health outcomes in this context (Popkin et al. 2012). Although there are some major critiques of the applicability of the nutrition transition model to all settings in time and space, the model provides a useful starting point from which to understand overarching global health trends, such as the dramatic increase in chronic noncommunicable disease (e.g., cardiovascular disease and metabolic syndrome) and overweight and obesity. Despite the fact that the overall explanatory power of the model may be insufficient in many settings, the links between increased globalization, diet and lifestyle changes, and health outcomes cannot be denied. This book contributes to expanding the literature on the nutrition transition and enhances our understanding of how globalized practices (i.e., participation in the global market economy, dietary delocalization, etc.) influence nutrition-related lifestyle changes and how this impacts health in localized settings. Due to paucity in the literature regarding pregnancy health and the important implications that changes to the food environment have for maternal and child health, this book explores the ways in which the nutrition transition impacts prenatal dietary practices in the Monteverde Zone. In order to do this, I draw on the CBCA in anthropology and practice theory from the social sciences. The main characteristics of these frameworks (i.e., the emphasis on links between political economy, culture, biology, and practice) provide a concrete way to identify the specific impacts of the nutrition transition on prenatal health.

Chapter 4

Expanding the Nutrition Transition

THE CRITICAL BIOCULTURAL APPROACH

The CBCA emphasizes the dynamic, dialectical relationship between biology and culture, while acknowledging the importance of political-economic processes that shape human health (Zukerman and Martin 2016; Goodman and Leatherman 2011, 1998; Singer 2001, 1998; Singer and Claire 2003). This framework developed contemporaneously with the new biocultural synthesis (Goodman and Leatherman 1998), which began to push critically beyond the limits of traditional theoretical models in biological and cultural anthropology in order to build a bridge between the subfields, which became increasingly divided as more time passed since the early twentieth century, when Franz Boas had advocated for a holistic approach in anthropology (Borofsky 2002). Beyond Livingstone's (1958) influential work on sickle-cell trait in the 1980s, biological anthropologists started to critique the adaptationist paradigm, which dominated the subfields within physical anthropology over the preceding decades (Leatherman and Goodman 2011; Levins and Lewontin 1985). The adaptation model was critiqued for being too reductionist, and Levins and Lewontin (1985) argued that the relationship between humans and their environment should be viewed as dialectical and complex. The influence that humans continually have on their environment should be taken into account when understanding the intricate relationship between environmental stress and human biology. Running parallel to this critique were the views of psychologists and sociologists from the 1960s through the 1980s, which argued against the stimuli-centered stress model that emphasized life events as being the center of stress and responses in human biology (Ice and James 2012).

As anthropologists point out, Seckler's (1980) small but health hypothesis, which ultimately explained small-bodied Indian neonates as an adaptation to low energy environments, "alerted many to the political implications of their science, in this specific case, whether or not millions MMM [mild to moderate malnutrition] Indian children would receive food aid" (Leatherman and Goodman 2011, 31). However, there was still a lack of discussion of human agency (i.e., "the interested practice of real people" [Ortner 2006:16]) and its interaction with power dimensions and environmental stimuli. During the same time period (between the 1960s and 1980s), debates were occurring in the field of medical anthropology regarding the relationship between biology and culture, which was traditionally fragmented in practice (Sobo 2011; Singer 1998). The field of medical anthropology, fully recognized by the 1960s, has from its inception critiqued the biomedical model (Singer 1998). This contributed to the integration of the political economy of health model into the discipline, ultimately leading to critical medical anthropology by the 1980s (Singer 1998). Political economy of health emphasizes the point that adaptations occur in response to social stressors that are ultimately a manifestation of social structures contextualized within class and imperialist relations within the capitalist system (Baer 1982). Notably, Paul Farmer's (2005, 2001) work with tuberculosis and AIDS in poor resource settings, such as Haiti and Peru, shows that social oppression, through mechanisms like structural violence, creates a higher susceptibility to disease and lower likelihood for treatment and recovery. Adaptation or coping strategies are employed within these populations who have access to limited resources and must make difficult choices about how to use the resources they do have.

However, the "chasm" between biology and culture continued in the second half of the twentieth century and Goodman and Leatherman (1998) argued for a conceptual model that encompasses a more critical approach to biocultural research (Leatherman and Goodman 2011). Goodman and Leatherman recognized that the traditional studies using a biocultural model in anthropology merely linked biology and culture and lacked the cohesion necessary to understand complex nutritional inequalities found around the world. Recognizing the way that biology and culture are "dynamically linked," Levins and Lewontin (1998) assert, "What we label as a 'dialectical' mode of thought is a mirror of the actual history of things in the world which in their historical actuality acquire their real, but ever changing properties in concrete, but every changing contexts" (xiii). The dialectical relationship between biology and culture is a key conceptual feature of the CBCA because it moves beyond the recognition of a dichotomy between the two artificially constructed concepts and encompasses the complexity of the biocultural interaction. However, over the years there have been many definitions associated with studies that employ the critical biocultural approach (Wiley 2016; Fouts et al. 2012; Kaye 2012; Melby and Lampl 2011; Watkins 2009; Ulijaszek and Lofink 2006; Brewis 2003; Li 2003; Singer and Clair

2003; Goodman and Leatherman 1998; Perez-Escamilla et al. 1995; Wiley 1992; Baer 1990; Beyenne 1986). And, perhaps more commonly, researchers engaged in biocultural research haven't actually defined the term or orientation (Ferzacca 2012; Stini 1995; Melby and Lampl 2011; Goodman et al. 1988). Although political economy was always a central part of constructing studies in biocultural anthropology, it became more emphasized over time, developing into what Leatherman and Goodman (2011) call the "critical" biocultural approach. "The point is that people don't just end up rich or poor, sick or healthy, landed or landless. These all happen for reasons, and those reasons frequently lie upstream. If there is a single overarching theme to a political-economic perspective it is in focusing upstream on the intersection of forces which place people by the river and push them in" (33). Political economy focuses on the role that social structures play in providing access to resources within and between populations. The emphasis is on factors related to social structures, such as the economy, policies, education and employment, among others. For example, Horton (2009) shows that the effects of ecotourism reinforced socioeconomic hierarchies in Costa Rica's Osa Peninsula, as efforts at conservation ultimately pushed out impoverished people living in the area. Further, while ecotourism is lauded for its strong ties with conservation and promotion of sustainable practices, those who most benefit already have economic and social capital to do so, calling to question ideas about "sustainability." Ecotourism has brought an economic boom to the Osa Peninsula, but individuals and groups that had historically lower economic and social capital work long hours for low pay, which shifts familial and social structures.

Goodman and Leatherman (1998) identified five interrelated issues that illustrate the way that political economy contributes to a biocultural studies: "the importance of examining biological variation in terms of social relations," "the importance of links between the local and the global (macro-micro interconnections)," "history and historical contingency," "humans are active agents in constructing their environments," and "ideology and knowledge, of subjects and scientists alike, are key to understanding human action" (19, 20). CBCA has been applied to a wide range of research within and across the subfields of anthropology (Lende 2005, 2012; McDade 2002; Blakely 1998; Morgan 1998; Armelagos and Goodman 1998; Hvalkof and Escobar 1998; Smith and Thomas 1998; Bogin 1995; Stuart-Macadam and Dettwyler 1995; Moffat 2001; Chavez et al. 1995; Carey 1990). But more central to the theme here, proponents of CBCA have used it to explore health in Latin America (Piperata et al. 2011; Oths 1998; Carey 1990; Brewis 2003). Further, this perspective has been applied to studies exploring the interaction between tourism and health (Himmelgreen et al. 2013; Nagata et al. 2011; Leatherman and Goodman 2005; Daltabuit and Leatherman 1998;

Leatherman 1996), as well as women's reproductive health (Daltabuit and Leatherman 1998; Browner 1989; Beyene 1986). Although many of these articles do not explicitly embrace CBCA, the discussion regarding biocultural interactions are framed within the context of shifting political economy, or explore the power dimensions within these interactions.

The landmark study in anthropology that first drew links between tourism-driven development and health from a biocultural approach was Daltabuit and Leatherman's (1998) work in the Yucatan. Throughout this research, Daltabuit and Leatherman (1998) investigated "how social and economic changes in the contexts of tourism development might be linked to biological changes in nutrition and health" (317) among Mayan households. Specifically, their work addresses household diet, nutrition, and health in the context of shifting gender roles, which they attribute to gender differences in illness. The authors found that increased workloads (associated with tourism) and reproductive stress led to poor health outcomes among women, and that the stress of being the head of the household may exacerbate this relationship. Building on this work, the "coca-colonization" described by Leatherman and Goodman (2005) refers to the tourism-related dietary shifts of the Mayan communities in the Yucatan and to the inclusion of and increased dependency on purchased foods as well as an increased consumption of processed foods, which are part of the industrial food system. This includes calorie-dense and nutrient-poor snack foods that begin to supplement the diet. In South America, Oths (1998) used the critical biocultural perspective to explore a biocultural model of the sickness process in the Andean highlands and found that "the observed health differences among Andean communities appear to be generated out of the unique confluence of ecological factors, local meaning and political-economic and historical processes which combine to shape systematic intra-Andean diversity" (1026). In line with the recommendations for the CBCA proposed by Goodman and Leatherman (1998), Oths emphasizes the multi-level analysis that contextualizes health within this community. Another feature of the CBCA involves exploring the links between the global and the local, which Carey (1990) emphasizes as he argues for an integrative approach using a biological and sociocultural perspective to understand morbidity in the rural Peruvian Andes. Carey's work argues for the adaptive health benefits of interhousehold social support networks within this community. The studies reviewed here clearly demonstrate the application of CBCA through their ability to link the macro with the micro, their exploration of biological variation within the different sociocultural contexts, their emphasis on historicity, and/or their emphasis on knowledge and ideology (Goodman and Leatherman 1998). While it makes sense that studies on health and well-being should take an approach that integrates both culture and various dimensions of human biology, this trend has only gained momentum over the last few decades. Further, the expansion of these analyses to include of macro-level forces, such as tourism-driven development, are even more recent.

Despite the contemporary expansion of the CBCA as a useful analytic model, most studies still fail to acknowledge the role of humans as active agents in shaping their environments. This is surprising, as Leatherman and Goodman (2011) have recognized that this perspective is essential to the CBCA. This book bridges this gap by applying an approach that emphasizes the role of human agency (i.e., "the interested practice of real people") (Ortner 2006, 16) in shaping women's prenatal dietary practices. Practice theory brings the focus of the discussion back to human agents and emphasizes their role in shaping community health in the face of constantly shifting environmental conditions brought on by a fast-paced globally connected society.

PRACTICE THEORY

"History makes people, but people make history" (Ortner 2006, 2). With the world growing smaller at an alarming rate, it is hard to keep up with the ways that macro-level processes actually affect local communities. More often than not, studies examining shifts in health over time do not adequately take into account the ways in which both biology and culture interact to produce change. Using the CBCA (Leatherman and Goodman 2011) as an umbrella, practice theory is used in this book to explore the ways that the nutrition transition has influenced prenatal dietary practices and nutritional status in the Monteverde Zone. There have been some attempts to contextualize the nutrition transition within local, lived realities (Abu-Saad et al. 2012; Kavle et al. 2017; Cantor et al. 2013; Dodd 2011; Piperata et al. 2011). However, I argue that practice theory makes a much-needed contribution to understanding the relationship between the nutrition transition and prenatal dietary practices and nutritional status, as well as to the application of CBCA overall. Even Leatherman and Goodman (2011) note that the application of the CBCA often lacks study of individual choice, behaviors, and accounts of human agency. Here, I will address this fragmentation by outlining the core tenets of practice theory and identify key aspects of this framework that can fill the gap in praxis when applying the CBCA and the nutrition transition to aspects of health and human well-being.

Ortner (2006) points out that there is no one unified vision of practice theory, although there is a core group of philosophers, academics, and theorists who have developed central concepts that have been woven together to form the fabric of this model. Most notably, this includes Erving Goffman, Anthony Giddens, Pierre Bourdieu, Marshal Sahlins, and Sherry Ortner (Ortner 2006; Sahlins 1981; Giddens 1979; Bourdieu 1977; Goffman 1959).

"The fundamental assumption of practice theory is that culture (in a very broad sense) constructs people as particular kinds of social actors, but social actors, through their living, on-the-ground, variable practices, reproduce or transform—and usually some of each—the culture that made them" (Ortner 2006, 129). Practice theory developed in the 1970s, when the major theoretical frameworks in the United States were theories of constraint, emphasizing the role of "external social and cultural forces and formations: by culture, by mental structures, by capitalism" (Ortner 2006, 1, 2). Surprisingly, this is still reflected in the application of the CBCA and the nutrition transition. Previous frameworks (i.e., functionalism, structuralism, symbolic anthropology, and Marxism) failed to take into account human agency or an acknowledgement of how constraints were produced and reproduced (Ortner 2006), although Geertz's symbolic anthropology did bring the focus onto the individual actors (Ortner 1984). Using micro-ethnographic techniques, the sociologist Erving Goffman (1967, 1959) studied interpersonal relations (i.e., symbolic interactionism and dramaturgy), bringing human agency into theory (Handler 2012). He also addressed game theory in his work, emphasizing "that interpersonal relations are a competitive game of status and prestige" (Knauft 1996, 113). However, Goffman almost entirely ignored structural constraints (Ortner 2006). In order to move beyond models of structure/agency opposition, Bourdieu, Giddens, and Sahlins all attempted to address the relationship between structure and agency. "They accomplished this by arguing, in different ways, for the *dialectical*, rather than *oppositional* relationship between the structural constraints of society and culture on the one hand and the 'practices'—the new term was important—of social actors on the other" (emphasis in original) (Ortner 2006, 2). Additionally, the post-structuralist practice theory embraced features of the Marxist perspective, acknowledging the facet of power within agency/structure interactions. This marked the difference between practice theorists and those who used an agency-oriented approach in their work. This transition and emphasis on critical analysis fits well with the trend in biocultural studies to include political economy.

Perhaps the most well-known of the group, Pierre Bourdieu's (1977) work is often synonymous with practice theory. Bourdieu draws on Goffman's discussion of strategy, involving status and prestige, and builds on this through his discussion of the role of various forms of capital in shaping subordination, which plays out through economic and symbolic inequalities (Knauft 1996). Bourdieu (1977) constructs the notion of "habitus," stemming from the work of Marcel Mausse and Durkheim, to form a construct of the "system" based on strategies or dispositions, as opposed to a pure notion of rules, as was developed by others, including Durkheim and his notion of social facts (Durkheim 1982), which created a system of constraint (Shusterman 1999). Bourdieu develops this construct further by explaining that the normalization of the arbitrariness of the system is what forms individuals' sense of reality and sense of limits. This occurs as the "habitus" engages in a dialectical relationship with the unconscious "systems of classification which reproduce, in their own specific logic, the objective classes, i.e., the divisions by sex, age, or position in the relations of production, make their specific contribution to the reproduction of the power relations of which they are product, by securing the misrecognition, and hence the recognition, of the arbitrariness on which they are based" (Bourdieu 1977, 164). Bourdieu calls this *doxa*, which should be distinguished from concepts such as "orthodoxy" and "heterodoxy," which imply a conscious awareness of alternatives beliefs (Bourdieu 1977). Although Bourdieu and Ortner both rely on the idea of "games" as central to their version of practice theory, Ortner (2006) develops the idea of what she terms "serious games," which emphasizes cultural variability, as opposed to universality, and begins to fill some of the other gaps left by a critique of Bourdieu's work. Unlike Bourdieu, whose work reflects the abstract nature of the dialectical relationship between structure and agency and tends to leave out the behaviors and practices of real people, Ortner grounds her work in deep ethnography, being "critical of the ethnographic 'thinness' in many existing studies of disempowerment or resistance" (Knauft 1996, 109). Further, Bourdieu has been critiqued for not acknowledging, or accounting for historical change or transformation (Knauft 1996). In contrast, Ortner (1984) stresses the importance of historicity and asserts that practice theorists aim to explain "the genesis, reproduction and change of form and meaning of a given social/cultural whole" (149). Through Ortner's (2001) ethnographic work, she touches upon motivation, which is absent from Bourdieu's work. Further, Bourdieu stresses symbolic and economic inequality in his work, but fails to adequately address other forms of inequality, such as gender, sexuality, racism ethnocentrism, or nationalism (Knauft 1996). Bourdieu has also been criticized for his definition of structure, which is somewhat vague and abstract. Ortner's (2006) deviation from the traditional concepts surrounding practice theory is a useful tool, which I refer throughout the rest of the book. I argue that Ortner's constructs associated with practice can be operationalized in a way that lends itself to systematic data collection, and this framework makes sense in the context of filling gaps left by macro-level explanations of global health trends.

The construct of agency is extremely important to practice theory, although it was almost entirely explicitly absent from Bourdieu's work (Ortner 2006). Ahearn (2001) tries to create a starting point through which to understand agency and defines agency as "the socioculturally mediated capacity to act" (113). Ortner (2006) describes the traditional concept of agency as being focused on a Western, individualistic model, embodying the image of the heroic individual exerting agency as he/she is up against the system at large.

As Ortner (2006) states, "Nothing could be further from the way I envisage social agents, which is that they are always involved in, and can never act outside of, the multiplicity of social relations in which they are enmeshed" (130). This is a key feature of this book, as there is an emphasis on the relationship between pregnant women and other social actors, as well as other forces that may (or may not) influence nutrition-related decision-making. This perspective allows Ortner (2006) to develop her construct of serious games, through which individuals are always involved with others, making it impossible for the agent to be free. As Ortner (1997) explains,

> The idea of the "game" is meant to capture simultaneously the following dimensions: that social life is culturally organized and constructed, in terms of defining categories of actors, rules and goals of the games, and so forth; that social life is precisely social, consisting of webs of relationship and interaction between multiple, shiftingly interrelated subject positions, none of which can be extracted as autonomous "agents"; and yet at the same time there is "agency," that is, actors play with skill, intention, wit, knowledge, intelligence. (12)

This view of agency will enhance the application of the CBCA to understanding the implications of the nutrition transition on prenatal dietary practices by accounting for the human capability to act in strategic ways and with intention, which is ultimately embedded in a specific sociocultural context in the Monteverd Zone. Using this as an analytic framework provides detailed information about maternal decision-making during pregnancy under circumstances that may promote food insecurity. Ortner's (2006) construct of serious games provides a framework for understanding the relationship between interrelated subject positions and intentionality in human agency, and through participant observation this exposes the ways that the rules of the game are intentionally followed or broken. There are two sides to the coin of serious games: one is solidarity in the "social embeddedness of agents" (130) and the other is that the "agent is always enmeshed within relations of power, inequality and competition" (131). I agree with Ortner that agency involves intentionality, which ultimately separates it from the notion of routine practices, or what Bourdieu refers to as *doxa*. Agency is both universal, as a feature of humanity, and distinct in that it is always historically, socially, and culturally constructed. Both power and intentionality are the two facets of agency, which include "(the pursuit of) 'projects' or as (the exercise of or against) 'power'" (Ornter 2006, 139). Cultural projects involve desires and goals that are cultural constituted, such as getting married. I apply the concept of cultural projects to the experience of pregnancy, as women in this study have interests in the survival of their offspring, but there are other actors who have a stake as well, including mothers, mothers-in-law, and partners.

Practice theory fills a large gap that no macro-level population studies of the nutrition transition can fill. Accounting for individual and group agency in the context of shifting environments will help to account for the way that the "system" is changing. This will connect the social changes occurring in the Monteverde Zone with the recent increased tourism and the nutrition transition.

LINKING PRACTICE THEORY AND THE CRITICAL BIOCULTURAL APPROACH

While I have already noted that proponents of the CBCA recognize the need for agency-oriented approaches in biocultural research (Leatherman and Goodman 2011), and that practice theory can fill that gap in the literature, it is important to outline both the strengths and the challenges of integrating the two frameworks.

Overall, practice theory adds to studies that use the CBCA by providing a well-established framework for applying an agency-oriented approach to this body of work. Practice theorists have long discussed and debated the role of human agency in regard to the ways that humans interact with their environments (Ortner 2006, 1984; Ahearn 2001; Goffman 1967, 1959). While studies that employ the CBCA do a good job at describing the ways that biology and culture interact in various settings and under shifting environmental conditions (Nagata et al. 2011; Oths 1998; Leatherman 1996), many fail to go beyond the "description" of these phenomena. An agency-oriented approach allows the researcher to produce a more in-depth analysis and identify the ways that individuals and groups make decisions within different contexts of environmental change, which ultimately leads to the outcomes being described by CBCA researchers. Finally, by using an agency-oriented approach to understanding decision-making in the context of shifting environments, and by drawing on firsthand data, this approach can contribute to health promotion efforts. A major challenge for health promotion is behavior change through successful implementation of intervention and prevention strategies (Wallace et al. 2014; Damschroder et al. 2009). While the application of practice theory doesn't necessarily fix this problem, it does provide a realistic framework as a starting point (i.e., understanding decision-making regarding health behaviors and collecting accounts of actual behaviors or practices).

While these strengths certainly add to the CBCA, there are also numerous challenges to applying a practice theory approach. First, as mentioned previously, there is not a unified version of practice theory (Ortner 2006). This has been a considerable barrier to standardizing methods and analysis, and may be one reason why this approach has not been more widely applied to studies using the CBCA. For this study, a mixed methods approach was used, which relied heavily on qualitative analysis using specific constructs from the practice theory literature. These data were quantified by examining the number of times each construct appeared in the narrative, as well as the number of times these constructs overlapped with others and the strength of association of those overlaps. Another challenge is the in-depth cultural knowledge required by researchers to successfully apply this model. For example, this book explores prenatal dietary practices and changes in constructs of human agency over time. In order to understand how pregnant women made decisions surrounding these practices, it was essential to develop a baseline description of what these practices were. This process was facilitated by my previous research in the area, as well as my cultural knowledge base that was developed over seven years and through repeated visits to the region. The other major challenge to applying this approach within the CBCA is the time needed to collect the data and conduct the analysis. In order for findings to be generalizable, the researcher has to make a sufficient number of firsthand observations. This includes not only a large enough sample size but also enough repeated observations of the same or similar phenomenon (e.g., decision-making surrounding a specific dietary practice, such as food cravings during pregnancy). Not only can this pose a challenge for researchers but it also places a high burden on participants, who need to agree to allow the researcher to spend significant amounts of time with them, as situations that the researcher needs to observe may not occur at predictable intervals. Analysis of the data can also be time-consuming, as there are various procedures for applying the practice theory approach, although none of which are tailored for biocultural research. I argue that streamlining some of the ways that practice theory is applied, such as the methodology described in this book, can improve implementation.

BRINGING IT TOGETHER: THE CRITICAL BIOCULTURAL APPROACH AND THE NUTRITION TRANSITION

From the CBCA, the major strength of the nutrition transition model is its engagement with globalization and political economy in order to explain shifting global health trends. Extensive research by Popkin (Popkin and Reardon 2018; Popkin 2015, 2012, 2004, 2002, 1994; Popkin et al. 2012, 1993; Drewnowski and Popkin 1997) links global practices, such as shifts in technology, prevalence and reliance on mass media, and dependence on the transnational food system, with specific changes in nutrition and increased rates of overweight and obesity, as well as other chronic noncommunicable diseases (e.g., cardiovascular disease, metabolic syndrome, type 2 diabetes, and hypertension). There is also a growing body of literature that links the nutrition transition with neoliberal trade policies that shift access and availability of nonlocal consumer goods and services (including food), which transform local economies and traditional systems of food production (Friel et al. 2013; Thow 2009; Thow and Hawkes 2009; Hawkes and Thow 2008; Rayner et al. 2006). For example, the North American Free Trade Agreement led to increased imports of soybeans, corn, sugar, snack foods, and meat products to Mexico, and similar outcomes have resulted from the Central American Free Trade Agreement in 2006 (Friel et al. 2013). This trade agreement that involves the United States, Costa Rica, El Salvador, Nicaragua, Honduras, Guatemala, and the Dominican Republic, with United States being the largest trade partner by far (Hicks et al. 2014; Koehler-Geib and Sanchez 2015). Forty-five percent of Costa Rican exports go to the United States and 45 percent of imports to Costa Rica are from the United States. In contrast, only 5 percent of imports come from Central America and 16 percent of exports are supplied to these local partners (Hicks et al. 2014). This has affected local access and availability of certain foods. For example, Costa Rica now imports the majority of beans from Nicaragua (in addition to Argentina and China through other trade agreements) (Arias 2014). A change in agricultural strategies in Nicaragua led to a bean shortage in the country in 2014 and has disenfranchised many local producers who cannot compete with the market (Arias 2014). Although Costa Ricans consume 4,100 tons of beans per month, less than 20 percent are now produced in the country, with 99 percent of red beans and 50 percent of all other beans coming from Nicaragua (Arias 2014). While Popkin and Reardon (2018) have recently questioned the roles and responsibilities of the multinational food industry, exemplified through corporations such as McDonald's and Coca-Cola, overall application of the model has steered clear of critical inquiry. The underlying power dimensions and hegemonic forces that shape policy decisions and influence global practices are largely ignored. In addition, the implications of these changes are framed as consequences of the implemented large-scale political-economic policies. While this is true to an extent, the response within local communities is largely ignored.

In chapter 3, I outlined the characteristics of the nutrition transition and described the health impacts of this global shift in the food environment. I also illustrated the ways that this framework can be expanded, by linking this macro-level phenomenon with the local reality of living in rural Costa Rica. Here, I situated the CBCA in anthropology in both historical and contemporary context, and identified the gaps in this framework for understanding decision-making and the role of humans as active agents of change at the community-level. These core concepts will be used throughout the rest of the book to better understand how a culturally situated framework regarding prenatal diet (i.e., customs, beliefs, and everyday practices) can inform global health promotion efforts.

RESEARCH DESIGN AND PRAXIS

Before moving on, I will briefly outline some of the relevant characteristics of the research design in order to link the theory with practice. The research on which this book is based[1] draws on the CBCA as a guiding theoretical framework (Leatherman and Goodman 2011), examining changing foodways in the Monteverde Zone from both a biological (i.e., dietary intake) and cultural (i.e., the human experience) vantage point, and exploring how the two interact and are intertwined. The examination of biological and cultural factors necessitated the use of a mixed methods study design, gathering data on quantitative (e.g., food insecurity status) and qualitative (e.g., women's narratives about dietary practices) measures. This investigation also took an applied and participatory approach, using methodology (i.e., participatory focus groups) that directly involved participants in identifying gaps in our knowledge and encouraged them to suggest solutions.

In light of the tourism-driven nutrition transition in the Monteverde Zone, I wanted to know, *how have increased tourism and the concomitant nutrition transition influenced prenatal diets and food-related practices in the Monteverde Zone?* In order to answer this question using a practice theory framework, it was also important to know as to *how have prenatal dietary practices shifted over the last generation, concurrent with the rise in tourism over the last twenty-five years?* In order to link these changes with potential impacts to health and human biology, I also asked, *what is the current nutritional status of pregnant women in the Monteverde Zone and what are the health implications associated with this status?* And, finally, in light of the high rates of food insecurity previously documented in the Monteverde Zone, it was also important to ask, *what is the relationship between food (in)security and prenatal nutritional status in the context of tourism and the nutrition transition?*

The methods and analysis used in this research directly answer these questions, while drawing on the CBCA and practice theory to guide the design and implementation of research. In order to explore the biological and quantitative dimensions of shifting dietary practices, twenty-four-hour recalls were used to assess nutritional status of pregnant women (n=21) and to identify the types of foods consumed and food sources. These data were triangulated with food security data (n=20), collected using the Household Food Insecurity and Access Scale (HFIAS), to assess the relationship between nutritional status and food security. Women's narratives were collected using semi-structured interviews (n=42) to document the experience of women living in this region. Interviews conducted with pregnant women (n=22) were compared to interviews with women with older children (children older than fifteen) (n=20) to explore changes in prenatal dietary practices and decision-making over time. These data[2] were triangulated with participatory focus groups (N=2, n=15) to assess women's attitudes about prenatal nutrition in the Monteverde Zone today. Free lists (n=52) were conducted to situate prenatal dietary practices within the context of culturally constructed ideas about nutrition. Participant observation was also used and provided insight to the ways that ideas about nutrition are actually put into practice.

NOTES

1. This study was approved by the Institutional Review Board (IRB) at the University of South Florida (#00017569) and preapproved by the Monteverde Institute, the local ethical body responsible for proper conduct of research involving human subjects in the Monteverde Zone.
2. All participants provided written or verbal informed consent prior to participating in the study. Pregnant women and older women provided written consent with the exception of women who had trouble with literacy. Survey participants provided verbal consent.

Chapter 5

Customs

¿Quiere un café? (Do you want some coffee?) Melissa asked me as she showed me to her kitchen table. I arrived in the early afternoon just in time for the *hora de café* (i.e., coffee hour). As Melissa was preparing the water to boil, it started to rain and I could see the thick white clouds roll over the banana plants and the other crops that were visible from the kitchen window. The cow figurines on her shelf peered down at me and their white bodies stood in stark contrast to the varying shades of blue that covered the grainy wood that constructed the house. As I heard the rain pattering on the roof I thought about the benefits of having a designated time every day dedicated to sitting down with others and sharing some food and slow conversation (i.e., *hora de café*). I also thought about how widespread this practice was in Costa Rica, making it a representative part of their culture, akin to the *siesta* in Spain (Javier 2015).

In addition to coffee, Melissa offered me a *chorreada*, not to be confused with *café chorreado* mentioned earlier. She explained that the *chorreada* was like a pancake, but made with *elote*, or corn straight from the cob. Melissa explained that *chorreada* was very simple and that the only ingredient was *elote*. She served the *chorreada* with *natilla*, the Costa Rican version of sour cream, made with the *nata*, or the creamy part of the cow's milk. Melissa's house was located amid a farming community and she and her family still relied on seasonal agricultural products, like *elote*. Unlike the seasonality associated with some foods in this rural community, *chorreada* is found all year round throughout Costa Rica. I found myself thinking of sitting in Melissa's wood farmhouse watching the clouds roll through while I ate *chorreada* in the central market in San José among the bustling stalls of vendors. I've also seen *chorreadas* on the menu at some *sodas típicas* (i.e., restaurants that serve typical Costa Rican foods) such as *gallo pinto* (breakfast dish consisting of rice and beans) and *casados* (a lunch dish consisting of rice and beans served with a protein and a salad).

After spending my first few months in Costa Rica, it was abundantly clear that most *sodas* serve the same foods with little variation. There seemed to be consensus on which dishes are inherently "Costa Rican." While many factors contribute to these shared ideas over time, one thing was clear: these dishes have come to be ubiquitous because of their popularity, their inextricable links with national identity, and the role of "customs" in shaping shared ideas about food and nutrition. The Monteverde Zone is no exception. There are particular customs that characterize dietary practices in the Monteverde Zone (like much of Costa Rica) and these *costumbres* are rooted in shared socio-cultural norms. As one of my participants noted, "Well, in Costa Rica we are always accustomed to eat rice, beans and meat, rice, beans and something. Always rice and beans" (Maricella, 25, 3 months pregnant). Diet also reflects the way that individuals and groups construct their identity. Another one of my participants explained that the customs of people are very important. She said, "Yes, or some because of customs. A mix of people has been created here [in the Monteverde Zone], from the city and from rural areas. And so, most are going to buy everything [i.e., food] and then there are others who go by their customs. But it's the rural farmers, *we* have the same food habits, and that's it" (Samantha, 60). At the heart of both of these sentiments is the idea that there are unspoken norms that guide food preferences. In order to better understand how this part of Costa Rican culture influences prenatal dietary behaviors in the context of the tourism-driven nutrition transition, I set out to define nutrition as a cultural context in the Monteverde Zone.

NUTRITION AS A CULTURAL CONSTRUCT

In order to identify shared ideas about nutrition, I used the concept of a semantic or cultural domain, which "may be defined as an organized set of words, concepts, or sentences, all on the same level of contrast, that jointly refer to a single conceptual sphere" (Weller and Romney 1988, 3). This method is particularly useful for defining a cultural domain in order to identify the boundaries of a domain in a specific cultural context (Weller and Romney 1988). In this case, I chose the concept of *la alimentación. La alimentación* means nutrition or nourishment and is extremely important to understanding food choices, as one can *alimentarse bien* ("eat well") or *alimentarse mal* ("eat poorly"). A free listing technique is often used to define a particular cultural domain (Weller and Romney 1988). Free listing has been used to explore various aspects of nutrition, such as basic knowledge (Shepard Jr. et al. 2008; Nebel et al. 2006), the transmission of cultural knowledge (Powell et al. 2014), to identify factors that influence food decision-making (Machin et al. 2014), and to explore attitudes toward specific foods or food categories (Muller and Almedom 2008; Roos 2002). In order to get at the cultural domain of *la alimentación,* I asked a random sample[1] of fifty-two people to list the factors that contribute to *la alimentación.* Gathering information on nutrition as a cultural domain helps to contextualize data on decision-making in relationship to the tourism-driven nutrition transition occurring in the Monteverde Zone. Free listing data was triangulated with interview data (n=42)[2] and focus group results (N=2, n=15) to broadly outline cultural consensus around nutrition in the Monteverde Zone. Overall, participants described the consumption or avoidance of specific foods, an understanding of the relationship between health and nutrition, the role of education in shaping nutrition, and the influence of the economy.

Food and Culture

"Yes, well, the usual. There was always vegetables, rice, beans, these things were never missing from the table of the Ticos, and they were always accompanied with something, with meat or chicken. That is, everything. Fruits too" (Lucía, 45). While Lucía was describing a traditional diet as she experienced it over time, Ticos today shared these ideas about what constitutes a typical diet. For free list participants, the most frequently mentioned food items that contributed to overall nutrition were fruits (e.g., watermelon), vegetables, and rice, and participants identified rice, beans, fruits, vegetables, salads, fish, balanced grains, food items with fiber, seafood, and milk as contributing to good nutrition. Since this region has traditionally relied on subsistence agriculture, fruits and vegetables have always been an important part of the diet, although the specific types of fruits consumed may be changing. Data from participant observation showed that this included items such as apples grown in other countries (e.g., Chile) and kiwis, which are available all year round, albeit for a high price. Other store-bought food items have been part of the diet since before there were formal roads in the region, prior to the arrival of the Quakers in 1951. Some older women in the sample remember riding on horseback to other communities so that they could purchase rice, beans, and other dried goods before there was a road in the area.

Maricella's earlier sentiment, "always rice and beans," reflects a shared sentiment with Lucía's understanding of what foods constitute a typical Costa Rican diet. When asked to define the domain of *la alimentación*, or nutrition, almost a quarter of free list participants responded with "rice and beans." Rice and beans is a dish that dominates meals in Costa Rica, and many places in Central America. In the morning, *gallo pinto* is often served for breakfast. Consisting of day-old white rice pan-fried with vegetable oil, sweet red pepper, onion, and cilantro, and served with eggs, tortillas, and cheese, this dish is a symbol of national pride. Although the actual origin of the dish is unknown, Costa Rica and Nicaragua both claim it as their own, which is often a point of contention due to the complex relationship between the two countries (Preston-Werner 2009). A typical lunch dish called *casado* consists of rice and beans served with a piece of meat (chicken, beef, pork, or fish), small cabbage salad with lime as a dressing, and cheese or a tortilla. Traditionally, in this region dinner would also consist of rice and meat, and possibly beans.

Some free listing participants identified junk foods a factor that contributes to poor nutrition, and among interview participants there was also a lot of discussion surrounding the term "comida *chatarra*," or "junk food," in relationship to dietary changes in the zone and poor nutrition. One pregnant woman explained that "junk foods" are street foods. She said, "How can I explain it to you, like street food. Hamburgers, fried chicken, things like that, foods that have a lot of fats are the ones I avoid" (Sofía, 22, 7.5 months pregnant). Another said that she received advice about these kinds of foods and that people told her, "Don't eat junk foods because they will produce a lot of saturated fats in your body and it won't provide nutrition to your baby, right" (María, 18, 6 months pregnant)? When talking about her kids, one older woman noted, "You give them cash so they can eat something and then they buy chips, Coca-Cola and other things like that. Then they have problems with gastritis. They don't eat food, or nutritious food, but they only eat foods like junk foods, because that's what they call it, junk foods. Then that is what makes them so sick" (Angelica, 44). Another women with older children commented about the effects of processed foods. She explained that her mother-in-law gave her some examples of why processed food is bad. She said,

> My mother-in-law isn't a doctor or makes decisions because of popularity, but she had a condition. She would tell me, "the color of a carrot is normal. If you put your finger inside carrot juice and it stays red, that is normal." But she told me, "do that with a packaged drink." It's a very strange test, right? She told me, "do it to see," she told me. Moisten your finger and put it in a package of powdered drink mix and your finger is going to stay that color. "That is what is going to your stomach." My mother in law never liked the powdered packages of Tang or any of those flavors. (Abigail, 41)

Similar to free listing respondents, interview respondents recognized that certain foods contributed to poor nutrition and were therefore bad for health. Interview participants were knowledgeable about the negative impacts of these foods. As one pregnant woman noted, "At least you know that soda has a lot of sugar, so you shouldn't consume too much" (Marina, 25, 6 months pregnant). This type of information was also passed down through the family. For example, one woman with older children noted, "Grandma always told me not to consume too much salt or fats and to avoid too much sugar. She was the only one who told me that" (Alma, 41).

Health

When asked to define nutrition, some free list participants defined this domain as a physiological need of the body (i.e., the body requires nutrients and energy) or made the connection between nutrition and *salud* (health). Free list participants also linked overall nutrition and having good nutrition with good health. They noted that the desire "to be healthy" and to "watch one's weight" was a driving factor to have good nutrition. Some interview participants spoke about the relationship between nutrition and health in terms of negative health impacts of poor nutrition, or how to improve health through nutrition. They also talked about this in relation to pregnancy. As one participant stated, "Ok, for example, if you eat a food that is going to give you diarrhea or something like that, it's a problem because during pregnancy you cannot take medicine. If there is a medicine, or a food that makes you sick, because of your pregnancy, you are not going to be able to take medicine. So, for example, with the flu or something similar, in general you can try to drink a lot of things with vitamin C and things that help you to avoid the flu/cold" (Maricella, 25, 3 months pregnant). Not surprisingly, pregnant women frequently talked about consuming a healthy diet for the health of their babies. For example, one pregnant woman said, "Similarly, after the baby is born I am going to try and eat healthy things so that she is okay because it also affects her health. Because if I am eating fried foods for lunch or something similar, that is what she is going to eat. So, it also affects her" (Rebecca, 21, 8.5 months pregnant). Weight was also a concern for pregnant women, as some were told by their doctors that they were gaining too much during their pregnancy. In contrast, only one woman with older children mentioned weight during narrative about diet and nutrition.

It's not surprising that people from the Monteverde Zone have a strong sense of the connection between diet and biological health. The average number of years of education (primary to tertiary) is fifteen and the literacy rate is 97.8 percent (Central Intelligence Agency 2019). In the Monteverde Zone, education is very accessible. This small community of approximately 6,000 people is home to public schools, two private schools (preK–12), a campus for a remote Costa Rican university, a Spanish language institute, and three institutions that offer programs in higher education to international students. Beyond identifying the links between diet and nutrition, there was also a shared understanding of what influences this relationship. Most commonly, participants mentioned factors associated with "dietary quality," which includes macro or micronutrients consumed or reference to having a balanced diet and avoiding junk foods or unhealthy foods and economic factors, such as reference to the economy in general, as well as individual income and the price of food. Some participants also mentioned "individual food items" such as fruits (e.g., watermelon), vegetables, and rice, or "factors related to health," such as the desire to be healthy, or in relation to things like disease, weight, or having a healthy digestive system.

Education

Free listing participants indicated that there was a link between education and both good and poor nutrition, and talked about the role of education and access to information. In contrast, interview participants were not forthcoming with a link between education and nutrition. When a few were probed about how they perceived prenatal diet in the Monteverde Zone today, they indicated that there was a relationship among education, family, and health. For example, one pregnant woman noted, "It really depends on the education of the family, right? And education, in my opinion, is also necessary because if there is a young girl of 14 years that ends up pregnant in a family without a lot of resources, this is a big problem" (Rosalinda, 31, 4 months pregnant). Another woman with older children noted, "Because when my daughter was little, she . . . I would give her nutritious foods here (at home), but in school she had bad nutrition. But now the government stopped that, the Ministry of Education stopped allowing the schools to have small eateries because the eateries have sweets and packaged foods" (Alma, 41).

Economy

Free listing participants indicated that economy affects nutrition (n=15), good nutrition (n=6), and poor nutrition (n=7) in the Monteverde Zone. There was consensus throughout interview narratives that food in the Monteverde Zone is very expensive. This was attributed to the tourism economy and dietary delocalization. Participants were aware that businesses raised their prices for tourism, as they believed that tourists had the money to spend, but also understood that most of their food comes from outside of the zone. When discussing tourism, one woman with older children explained. "Yes, I think because we are a tourist zone the business owners think that everything should be more expensive because there is a lot of money, but it's a little bit difficult for those of us who are from here and we don't have, we don't have enough resources to pay a lot, right" (Emma, 52). When a pregnant woman was probed about the high price of rice she noted, "Almost everything, yes, because all of the food comes from far away outside of the zone, so the rice too" (Estela, 25, 2.5 months pregnant). Another pregnant woman who lives in an agricultural community explained that because of the high prices it was sometimes hard to purchase enough for the whole family. She went on to say,

> Maybe, but not completely, but it [economic factors] influences it a little bit, because, well, we know that we have to buy a certain quantity because we are four, so if I want to buy something I have to think that I'll have to buy a high quantity because everyone is going to want to eat the same. Or something to drink. So, yes, I think that economic factors influence it, especially in that sense. Depending on the amount I would need to buy, so yes, it's harder. And, especially harder here in the zone. Okay, in Santa Elena there are more options and different places, where there are different prices or accessibility to buy cheaper vegetables because the same people in the zone can cultivate them for cheaper. But, it's already harder to get up to Santa Elena, going up to bring them down. The quickest option is the convenience store [nearby], which is more expensive. (Maricella, 25, 3 months pregnant)

In contrast, another woman living in an agricultural community stated, "Like for salads, yes, it's more expensive, because the tomato is more expensive. Or, to eat fruits. It's the same, a lot of fruits are very expensive. So it's hard. Okay, because I live in *El Valle*[3] there are a lot of fruits and vegetables that grow here. So, thank goodness you don't have to buy that much" (Rebecca, 21, 8.5 months pregnant). While most participants relied on store-bought foods items, some interview participants indicated that they buy some items when they leave the zone, since there are more options and food in general is less costly. Many women in the sample did not leave the zone specifically to purchase food, but took advantage of the low food costs when they left for other reasons (e.g., to attend school or visit family), although there were a few women who indicated that it was cheaper to go to Las Juntas (an hour and half bus ride) and do shopping for the month than stock up in Santa Elena. There was also recognition that the cost of food was high and was directly related to tourism. For example, some women noted that meat was more expensive when the tourist season was low. Local farmers set their own prices against those of the grocery store (i.e., the market) so when the tourism season goes down meat prices rise everywhere in the zone. As one pregnant woman discussed the effects of the low tourist season on her husband's paycheck she said, "Yes, it has a big impact because it's true: before I didn't eat as much packaged meats like now because they are cheaper" (Caroline, 24, 6.5 months pregnant). Another pregnant woman discussed the links with the tourism industry and explained that if tourism goes down, "then it cuts a bit, it cuts a bit into the economy of the house, you have to cut costs and you have to reduce what you eat because there is not enough to spend, the money is not enough to buy the nutritious foods that you should buy" (María, 18, 6 months pregnant).

Participants knew that on the weekends the grocery stores lowered their prices, but complained that the hotels would arrive early and buy all the good quality food. Through participant observation it was also clear that there was a differential effect of economic factors on food access depending on how far women lived from town. Women who needed to take a taxi to Santa Elena explained that it could cost 5,000 colones (almost $10) each way just to get to the store, in addition to the cost of food. Some even indicated that economic factors weighed more heavily on costs associated with transportation, doctor visits, and children's needs (diapers, formula, etc.) than on diet and/or nutrition.

Focus Groups

Participatory focus groups were conducted with mothers of varying ages in two distinct communities in the Monteverde Zone. One community was heavily rooted in agricultural and was approximately thirty minutes from the downtown area of Santa Elena. The other community was centrally located and is a short, walkable distance to goods and services that were centrally located near downtown. Although focus groups have roots in marketing (Bernard 2006), they are commonly used in other disciplines such as anthropology and public health. These workshops were based off of a participatory action research format that has been widely used in Peru and Bolivia to explore various women's health issues (Hammer et al. 2004). This included various activities and discussion. As one feature of participatory approaches is to break down the power dynamics between the researcher and the respondents, participant responses and discussion points were validated through researcher's note-taking. During each focus group, participants engaged in an icebreaker activity where they listed their favorite food. Subsequently, women participated in two activities with a short discussion that followed. During the first activity mothers were asked to identify factors that contribute to nutrition. Then they were asked to identify barriers to good nutrition. This activity was done as a group. During the second activity participants were asked to get into smaller groups and map their communities, including roads, bridges, houses, health posts, schools, places of worship, government organizations, plazas, informal markets, stores, agricultural land and use, bodies of water, etc. They were asked to identify the three most important resources for prenatal nutrition and explain why.

Focus group participants listed similar factors when asked about what influences nutrition. In the agricultural community, participants indicated that *costumbres*, or customs, were a major influence on nutrition. The group went on to clarify that it's actually the Costa Rican customs, or *costumbres Ticas*, such as the *hora de café*, that really dictate dietary behaviors and overall nutrition. When probed about factors that contribute to nutrition, women also listed other things such as stages of life (e.g., the prenatal period), what was available in the house, economic factors, and the distance from food resources, such as the supermarkets in Santa Elena. In contrast, the focus group closer to downtown said, having knowledge about what to eat, food groups, having variety, eating food with nutrients your body needs, having a balanced diet, making smart decisions, the amount of foods (e.g., sugar and fats), hydrating yourself, and the color of the foods (e.g., eating something green). When asked about limitations to good nutrition, women in the agricultural community responded as follows: not having supermarkets in their area, lack of transportation (e.g., having to wait for public transportation to get to a supermarket), there shouldn't be barriers to accessing good nutrition, not drinking water, habits, prices, accessibility, customs, and not having a home garden. In contrast, the group near downtown said, food groups (e.g., eating too much fat), customs that you develop when you are young, depends on each person (i.e., their body, education, and experiences), lessons learned about nutrition, it's hard to change, education, depends on the country, genetics, work (e.g., if you work in tourism it can change your eating patterns), and economic factors (e.g., before people grew more food and now food is more expensive).

Interestingly there were key differences during the focus groups when women were asked to draw their communities and identify resources that influenced nutrition (see figures 5.1, 5.2, and 5.3). As you can see in the maps the women made, in the agricultural community, there was more variety in food sources and they listed specific food items.

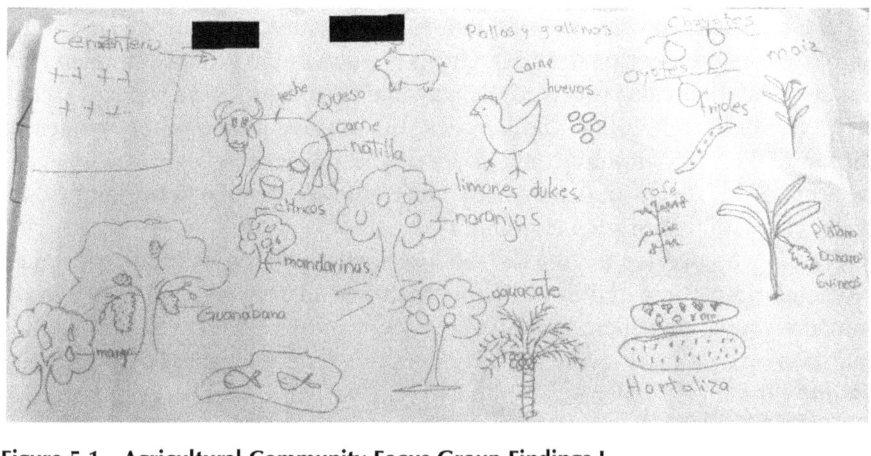

Figure 5.1 **Agricultural Community Focus Group Findings I.**

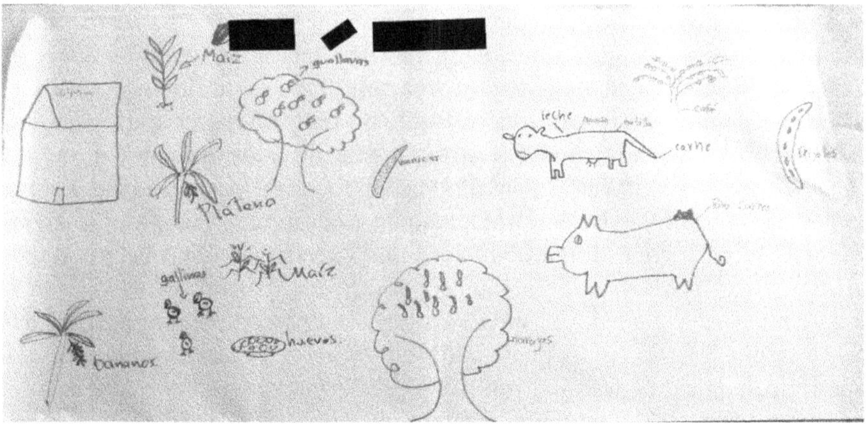

Figure 5.2 Agricultural Community Focus Group Findings II.

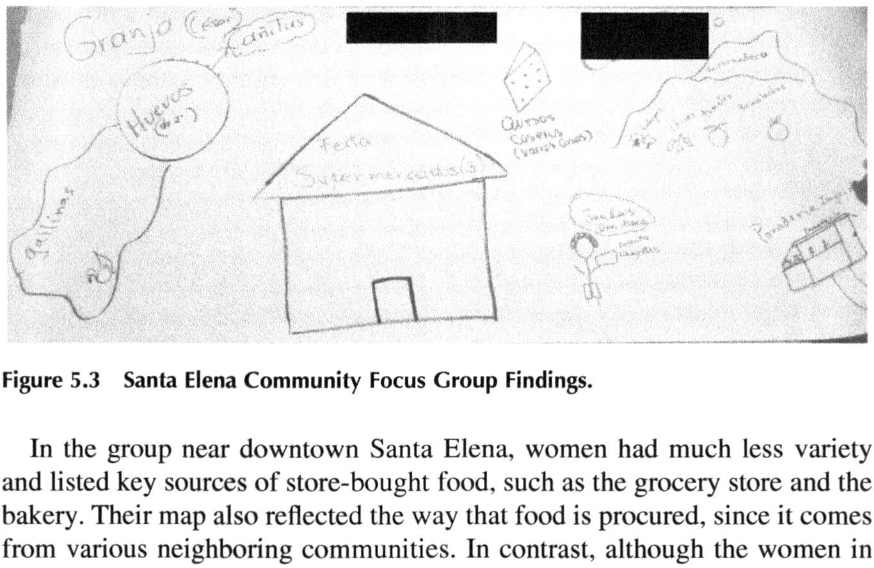

Figure 5.3 Santa Elena Community Focus Group Findings.

In the group near downtown Santa Elena, women had much less variety and listed key sources of store-bought food, such as the grocery store and the bakery. Their map also reflected the way that food is procured, since it comes from various neighboring communities. In contrast, although the women in the agricultural community talked about the distance to the grocery store as a major barrier to nutrition, they were able to identify many nutritional resources within their own community.

Clearly, the overlap among the random sample of free listing participants, women who participated in the semi-structured interviews, and focus group mothers shows that there is a shared understanding about what constitutes nutrition on a cultural level. Not only does this reflect aspects of Costa Rican identity, but it also reflects community characteristics, such as access to education, which influence how the tourism-driven nutrition transition is experienced at a local level. This type of in-depth analysis is exactly what Ortner

(2006) calls for in the context of understanding practice. Creating a cultural starting point helps to contextualize this community's experiences within a certain place and time. This lays the foundation for understanding how larger structural forces, such as the nutrition transition, directly and indirectly impact community health.

NOTES

1. Street-intercept surveys are considered a type of space sampling method (Lang et al. 2004). This methodology relies on geographic space to obtain a random sample when no sampling frame exists (Lang et al. 2004). Each individual that indicated they would participate provided verbal informed consent, confirmed that they were over eighteen years of age, and indicated that they were a local resident of the Monteverde Zone. In order to access a random sample, I stood on the street corner at one of four locations. The farmer's market and the three main supermarkets (Super Compro, Mega Super, and Super Vargas) were chosen as they are the main sources of purchased food (which fits with the theme of the study) and are located in public spaces with many individuals passing by regularly. The principal investigator stood at each location for one hour on a day chosen at random. An online random number generator (random.org) was used to produce specific dates for data collection.
2. The average age of free listing respondents (38 years) was similar to interview participants (35 years), indicating that data may be comparable across groups, as, on average, these individuals would have experienced the same structural changes that have occurred over time in the area, although perhaps in different ways.
3. Pseudonym.

Chapter 6

Cultural Beliefs and Everyday Practices

At first the road was empty. But, by the time I reached the end of the pavement where the dirt began, I saw a cluster of chickens running in front of a row of houses where someone was listening to *bachata* music. I peered into Cynthia's house and saw that the faded and scratched black leather couches were pushed to one side of the room to accommodate the baby shower decorations. Blue and green streamers were carefully hung on the wall amid paper cutouts, which were shaped to resemble babies and a pacifier. An elderly woman was sitting in one of the leather chairs and another middle-aged woman was in the kitchen cooking. A young woman sat with her nine-month-old baby and three young children ran around chasing each other. A few other women showed up as the party got started. The table in the center of the room had a white paper tablecloth and was adorned with plates of sweets: fruit flavored candies, different colored marshmallows on toothpicks and button-sized jelly candies covered in sugar. There was also a platter of crackers with tuna fish and chunks of corn and, of course, they served *arroz con pollo*, or rice with chicken. This dish is traditionally served on special occasions and is also ubiquitous to *sodas típicas* across Costa Rica. This main dish was served with a side of black refried beans from a bag and three Rumba-brand tortilla chips. As I moved the food around the plate with a fork, the grease smeared and glistened, creating a bright red contrast to the artificial white color of the plastic surface. The red tint to the grease was surely the *achiote* paste, which is a key ingredient to Costa Rican *arroz con pollo* and is made from achiote seeds, which are native to Latin America. In other regions this is known as annatto. While this scene of women and children sharing *arroz con pollo* at a baby shower certainly reflects shared ideas about Costa Rican culture and customs, I began to wonder what pregnant women meant when they continuously told me that their everyday diets were "*lo normal*" or, "the usual." When women were asked to describe their diet during semi-structured interviews, they commonly used this phrase. I wondered if delocalized dishes, such as *arroz con pollo* made with industrialized chicken, packaged bagged beans, and processed chips, had come to dominate everyday dietary practices, or if the experience I had at the local clinic and the woman's baby shower described here were abnormal. I also wanted to find out what the relationship was between these cultural practices and dietary health. In order to do this, I conducted forty-two semi-structured interviews with pregnant and nonpregnant women and identified local dietary practices that are associated with pregnancy. Embedded within these dietary practices are cultural beliefs that play a role in the relationship between decision-making, human agency, and change, which is described in the next chapter. I also collected dietary recall[1] information from pregnant women (n=21) to determine what they were "actually" eating. Twenty-four-hour diet recalls have been used to assess nutritional status during pregnancy cross-culturally (Ajantha et al. 2015; Park and Eicher-Miller 2015; Tijerina Sáenz et al. 2014; Ali et al. 2013; Castillo et al. 2011). With this information, I was able to draw links between the cultural construction of *la alimentación* (mentioned in the previous chapter as a cultural construct) and biological nutrition. Understanding the biocultural dimensions of changes in local foodways is paramount to identifying the impacts of the nutrition transition on prenatal health.

"LO NORMAL"

"*Lo normal*," or "the usual," was a common response among both pregnant and nonpregnant women when asked about their prenatal diet. Overall, pregnant women consumed a diet that included typical Costa Rican foods. The majority of women ate *gallo pinto* for breakfast, which was accompanied by eggs and in some cases processed meats (i.e., sausage, bacon, ham, or mortadella), farmer's cheese, fried plantains, tortilla, and/or sour cream. Further, the majority of pregnant women ate a dish of white rice and beans (either red or black) at some additional time during the day. This reinforces the idea that rice and beans were not just a part of the collective identity of Costa Ricans, but were also part of "actual" dietary practices. Women also ate fruits such as unripe mango, kiwi, bananas, and oranges, drank *frescos* (e.g., blackberry and *cas*), and consumed a variety of meats (e.g., fried pork, chicken, beef stew, and steak).

While nutritional status associated with actual dietary behaviors was adequate overall, saturated fat intake was high. Interestingly, some of the greatest contributors to saturated fat intake for all women were foods that were considered a normal part of the diet (e.g., chicken soup, rice pudding, sausage, and *empanadas*). Coffee was also part of this typical diet, and although participants noted that drinking too much caffeine was bad for health, three quarters of women drank coffee at least once a day on the day of the recall. Some drank coffee multiple times a day and some drank it sweetened with white sugar. Most women who drank one cup of coffee a day did so during the *hora de café* and also consumed a fatty or sugary snack (e.g., empanadas or sweet pancakes) during this time. This further highlights the influence of cultural practices on diet and behavior.

PRENATAL DIETARY PRACTICES

In addition to the clear links between what pregnant women perceive as a typical diet and Costa Rican customs, specific prenatal dietary practices rooted in the cross-cultural literature (Junges et al. 2014; Henrich and Henrich 2010; Lee et al. 2009; Christian et al. 2006; Sahoo and Panda 2005; Hartini et al. 2005; Phillips 2005; Izugbara 2003; Obeyesekere 1963) also emerged from women's narratives. This includes foods consumed because of health benefits, avoided foods, taboo foods, and food cravings. I compared these practices with women's experiences fifteen years ago or more, before the tourism boom and subsequent nutrition transition. These differences shed light on how changes to the food environment shape actual dietary practices during pregnancy today.

Food Consumed for Health Benefits

While the broader literature on prenatal diet points to examples of dietary prescriptions, pregnant women in the Monteverde Zone spoke more about consuming foods for health benefits, than for cultural reasons. Women talked about consuming foods for particular micronutrients (e.g., iron, fiber, potassium, calcium, and folic acid) or vitamins (e.g., vitamin C), or to help prevent a specific health problem (e.g., anemia, constipation, immune function, bone growth, regulation of blood sugar, muscle cramps, and vision) (see table 6.1). Anemia was a major concern for women and they indicated that eating specific foods would help with this (e.g., liver, beans, or green foods).

It's not surprising that women made connections between diet and biological health. Previously, I noted that literacy is high in Costa Rica and that education is particularly accessible in the Monteverde Zone. In addition, women received high levels of prenatal care during their pregnancies. All pregnant women in the sample attended monthly prenatal exams at the local clinic and took dietary supplements daily. Some women also received regular care from private obstetricians outside the Monteverde Zone. There was also the

Table 6.1 Foods Consumed for Benefits among Pregnant Women

N=20	
Food	*Reason for Consumption*
Liver	Anemia
Meat	Anemia/vitamins
Beans	Anemia/vitamins/iron
Green foods (e.g., spinach)	Anemia/iron
Coyote cilantro	Anemia
Red meat	Iron/nutrients for baby
Swiss chard	Iron/folic acid/vitamins
Fruits (kiwis, oranges, watermelon, melon, mango, mandarin oranges, orange rind, grapes, strawberries, avocado, orange rind)	Vitamins/clean skin (for PW)/Iron/ anemia/protein
Vegetables	Vitamins/clean skin (for PW)/iron/ anemia
Ripe plantain	Nutrients
Banana	Potassium to help with leg cramping
Cereals/oatmeal/cereals with fiber	Iron/constipation
Papaya/papaya juice	Digestion/constipation
Oranges, limes, and mangos	Vitamin C
Broccoli and eggplant	Immune function
Pineapple	Diuretic
Dairy (e.g., milk, yogurt, cheese)	Calcium/bone growth of baby/iron/acid reflux
Acidic lime	Regulate blood sugar/clean skin (for newborn)
Flaxseed or chia	Clean skin (for newborn)/help with birth
Legumes (e.g., lentils and garbanzos)	Clean skin (for newborn)
Apples	Clean skin (for newborn)
Fish	Vitamins
Rice	Vitamins
Chicken	Vitamins
Less processed foods	Have less hormones and less chemicals
Liquids/water/clean water	Avoid infection
Salads	No benefit specified
Beets	No benefit specified
Legumes	No benefit specified
Eggs	Protein
Grains	Iron
Nuts	Iron
Oil	Easy birth
Fresh orange juice	No benefit specified

preparation for birth class, which I have already described. During this three-day course women learn about women's rights in the hospital, oral health, lactation and breastfeeding, and taking care of their infant, among other things. The course is taught twice a year, and sometimes the clinic staff (i.e., physicians, nurses, oral healthcare professionals, and the resident psychologist) offer information about nutrition.

In addition, some foods were listed because pregnant women noted that they helped to give the mother and/or baby clean skin. While there was consensus that flaxseed could help with this, other responses varied, and included apples, lime, watermelon, fish, lentils, garbanzos, chamomile, avoiding cabbage, *mozote* (i.e., burgrass), and avoiding pineapple (and other acidic foods). As one participant indicated, "Yes, they are telling me to drink a lot of flaxseed, because this cleans the baby while it's still inside the stomach, and the baby will be born very clean. There are some babies that come out with white things and things stuck to their skin. So, that's it, when you drink flaxseed, they say that it cleans the baby" (Alejandra, 19, 8 months pregnant). Three women indicated that keeping their own skin clean was important and mentioned that staying hydrated, eating sweet limes, and consuming sour milk can help with this.

This idea was also associated with the hot/cold disease theory described later, as part of the reasoning behind avoiding "hot" foods was so that the baby would be born with *piel limpia*, or clean skin. This idea was not associated with any health implications, just the desire to have a newborn with clean skin.

In contrast to pregnant women, older women reported a larger variety of foods that were consumed because of benefits (63 vs. 50 food items). Although pregnant women linked specific foods with nutrition and health status, there were fewer items listed. Older women also listed more local and natural foods, reflecting the changes in dietary delocalization and food preference that have occurred in the region. For example, older women indicated that *yuplón* fruit, *anona* fruit, *cas*, *guineo negro*, guava, and sour sop are fruits that have benefits. These are locally grown fruits. In contrast, pregnant women listed items such as strawberries, kiwis, and grapes, which are not traditionally grown in this region but are more accessible now because of increased infrastructure and the dietary delocalization, which has occurred in the zone. Additionally, older women listed more traditional foods to the region, such as soups and foods such as squashes and *tacacos* (a native tree fruit).

Foods Avoided

There was a distinction made between foods that should be avoided for some reason and foods that are absolutely taboo and should not be consumed under any circumstance. Foods that should be avoided fell into one of three categories. First, there are foods that have harmful substances (see table 6.2). This includes hormones, chemicals, and caffeine. There was recognition that some meat, like chicken and fish, has harmful substances and should be avoided.

Table 6.2 Food Avoidances among Pregnant Women

N=19	
Food	*Reason for Avoidance*
Chicken in excess	Hormones
Tuna in excess	Hormones/mercury
Coffee	Caffeine
Soda	Caffeine/sugar
Unpasteurized dairy (e.g., milk and farmer's cheese)	Bacteria
Fats	Weight gain
Banana in excess	Weight gain
Fried pork rinds	Fats
Lard	Fats
Fried foods (e.g., fried chicken)	Fats
Fast foods/street foods (e.g., hamburger)	Fats
Junk foods (e.g., chips)	Fats/sugars
Mayonnaise	Salmonella
Sweets (e.g., chocolate, candies, ice cream, desserts, and honey)	Sugar/cause nausea
Salt in excess	Harmful
Oil in excess	Harmful
Food in excess	Harmful
Carbohydrates in excess (e.g., pasta, bread, and rice)	Harmful/refined carbohydrates
Sugars	Harmful
Undercooked or raw meats or seafood	Harmful/parasites
Packaged meats	Harmful
Condiments	Harmful

For example, chicken has hormones that can lead to rapid growth and development in humans and fish can contain mercury and hormones. Pregnant women also recognized the link between caffeine and certain beverages, such as soda and coffee.

Second, food safety was a concern for women. Pasteurization was something that was mentioned, as well as the distinction between raw and cooked meats/seafood. Unpasteurized milk was also something to avoid, along with locally produced unpasteurized cheese (i.e., farmer's cheese, or *queso fresco*) due to the bacteria these products can transmit. It is interesting to note that while women recognized these links, they still consumed farmer's cheese, which was a major contributor to saturated fat within the sample. Seafood and raw meats should also be avoided. Mayonnaise should be avoided because it contains raw eggs and can cause salmonella and pork needs to be cooked properly.

Finally, pregnant women mentioned foods with harmful macronutrients. This includes consumption of too many fats or carbohydrates. Pregnant women talked about trying not to eat junk foods or street foods because of their fat content, but also mentioned that too many fats (e.g., fried pork rinds and lard) were harmful. They noted that foods with too many carbohydrates (e.g., breads, flours, and fruits) could lead to weight gain. They also indicated that they should consume less salt, sugar, and oil in general. One participant noted that energy drinks, such as Maxx Energy can produce spina bifida and therefore should be avoided as well, although she did not provide a reason for this. Again, it's not a surprise that women linked food avoidances with specific health concerns as they had access to education and healthcare.

Although there were similar food avoidances reported for pregnant women and older women (e.g., fats, sugars, fried foods, salt, coffee, flour, and fast foods), there was an awareness about harmful substances in food and food safety practices by pregnant women that was not reported by older women. As mentioned previously, pregnant women discussed food avoidances in terms of harmful substances (e.g., caffeine or chemicals), food safety (e.g., pasteurization and bacteria from undercooked foods), and harmful macronutrients (e.g., too many fats or carbohydrates). However, older women provided few explanations for food avoidances, beyond mentioning that theywere harmful in general, causing stomach issues like gastritis (e.g., broccoli, cabbage, or lettuce), or being too acidic, with the consequence of damage to the baby's skin (e.g., pineapple). Pregnant women provided many explanations that were rooted in the medical model (e.g., the consumption of too many fats would lead to weight gain), representing the link between diet, nutrition and health, and possibly reflecting the influence of the local clinic. Overall, older women and pregnant women identified the same number of food items that should be avoided (20 vs. 21 food items).

Food Taboos

Food taboos (as distinguished from foods that should be avoided), fell into three groups: (1) abortive (i.e., will cause an abortion or miscarriage if consumed), (2) "hot" foods that have the potential to "burn" the baby's skin, and (3) other substances (i.e., alcohol and tobacco) (see table 6.3). There was also a hint of the belief in hot/cold dualities, where foods and beverages are classified as hot or cold and can have effects on health based on this knowledge (Messer 1981). In this study, items were only described as "hot" and no items were described as "cold." This idea was applied to two findings. First, this concept was applied to the idea that some teas are too hot for the body and can cause exudation of the baby (i.e., miscarriage or spontaneous abortion). These items were mostly teas such as chamomile and rosemary. Other items were considered abortive such as young coconut water and flaxseed. The explanation for most of these items is that they help with inflammation, and therefore consumption during pregnancy will cause your body to treat the baby as an infection and get rid of it. Additionally, cinnamon, mint, and rosemary teas are abortive because they are considered "hot" items and will relax the mother so much that the baby might come out.

Table 6.3 Food Taboos among Pregnant Women

N=13		
Abortive Substances (n=11)	*"Hot" Foods (n=7)*	*Other (n=4)*
Teas (chamomile, green tea, linden, rosemary, mint, and cinnamon)	Spicy foods (e.g., peppers and hot sauce)	Alcohol
Honey	Condiments	Tobacco
Red onion	Coca-Cola	Tea (unspecified) causes malformations
Pineapple		
Arracache (root vegetable)		
Crowned essence		
Young coconut water		
Flaxseed		

Second, this was the explanation for the taboo against consuming "hot" foods because they would "burn" the baby's skin since they are too hot and will leave the baby with red marks or splotches on their skin when they are born. This includes Coca-Cola, hot peppers (or anything spicy), condiments, and packaged foods (e.g., chips). As one participant said, "Born red, yes, I've heard that because my mother told me that. You shouldn't eat spicy peppers because the baby will be born red. Beliefs" (Rebecca, 18, 7 months pregnant).

Interestingly, some items that were not acceptable to consume during pregnancy, such as flaxseed and crowned essence, were recommended to consume close to the due date of the baby. These drinks help the birth process, making it easier, faster, and ensure the baby's skin will come out clean.

Food taboos were similar for both pregnant women and older women and consisted of categories mentioned previously; items that cause miscarriage or abortion and foods that "burn" the newborn's skin. It is worth noting that the list of taboo items was much shorter for older women than for pregnant women, reporting eight specific items, whereas, pregnant women listed seventeen items. These results are surprising since the other data show that pregnant women get information from their families, and that their mothers-in-law may be influential when it comes to prenatal dietary taboos. This could be a result of the small sample size. Or, it could reflect the ways that culture changes in relationship to the changes in the environment. For example, some pregnant women indicated that drinking soda during pregnancy could lead to *piel manchada* (hives or red splotches).

Food Cravings

Boca abierta (i.e., "open mouth") refers to the belief that women should always fulfill their food cravings while they are pregnant or their child will be born "wanting," with their mouth open. This means that the baby will always have cravings for food, or that the baby will have a lot of drool (i.e., mouthwatering). One woman with older children explained that she was told about this practice when she was pregnant. She said, "And, eat everything it is that you want to eat, because if not the baby is going to come out with his mouth open." She went on to explain,

> With the open mouth, I don't know, or he will come out drooling, spitting out a lot of drool if you don't eat, a lot of drool for a baby. I don't know if this is true or not. That's what they told you back then. If you weren't eating what your body was asking for, then the baby would come out with an open mouth and spitting drool because the baby would be wanting to eat something. (Angelica, 44)

Although some women indicated that they didn't fulfill their cravings simply because of this belief, all the women in the sample understood the reference and the meaning behind it. Food cravings also consistently fell into various categories for pregnant women. This included comfort foods, avoided foods, acidic foods, and typical or usual Costa Rican foods. Homemade items were commonly reported, such as a specific dish made by the woman's family (i.e., mother, grandmother, or sister). Pregnant women reported craving many items that were also listed as items to be avoided, such as sweets and fried foods. Acidic foods were also craved, such as lime with salt. Foods that are part of the local culinary tradition were also listed, such as *chamol* (root vegetable) and bean sprouts, and various fruits, such as *jocotes*, *mamón chino* (lychee), *manzana de agua* (Malay water apples), *guabas* (ice-cream bean fruit), and plantains. There were additional items listed that did not fit into these categories, and included Aztec soup and a Cesar salad. Additionally, these categories are not mutually exclusive, as many avoided food items, comfort foods, and acidic items are part of the typical local diet.

Similar to pregnant women, older women listed food cravings that could be grouped into the following categories: foods on the avoided list, acidic foods, and typical foods. However, they did not discuss comfort foods as part of their narratives. Interestingly, three foods that were craved were items that were listed as taboo, which included wine, spicy vegetables in vinegar (*chilero*), and hot peppers with onion and lime. Both pregnant women and older women listed items that were previously identified as foods that should be avoided, such as fried foods (e.g., fried pork), fast foods (e.g., hamburgers), and sweets (e.g., cake and ice cream). These findings indicate that while there may have been some changes in dietary preferences and intake over time in the Monteverde Zone, the presence of these junk foods in the diet is not new. Additionally, older women listed fewer items than pregnant women (42 vs.

59 food items). This could be a result of shifting food access (e.g., presence of supermarkets).

These differences show that prenatal dietary practices among this sample have changed over time, although in more modest ways than originally hypothesized. Older women listed more natural foods that were consumed for benefits than pregnant women, possibly reflecting a shift in food access. However, avoidances, taboos, and cravings were similar for both groups, highlighting the ways in which culture is embedded in dietary practices. Another noted difference is the ability of pregnant women today to provide more detailed explanations for these practices, as well as an increased awareness of food safety issues, such as health risks of unpasteurized dairy products. This could be a result of the continued presence of the clinic as a source of information.

DIETARY PRACTICES, THE NUTRITION TRANSITION, AND HEALTH

It is clear that actual dietary practices and perceptions about prenatal practices overlap but the question remains as to if the foods consumed by pregnant women are characteristics of the nutrition transition and what health impacts this may have. During the prenatal period women have specific nutritional needs that need to be met to ensure proper growth and development of the fetus, optimal long-term fetal health, and to meet the demands of the mother's regulatory and tissue functions during gestation (Ritchie and King 2008). Although women may need to make sure that they receive adequate energy during the first trimester to support their fetus, nutritional requirements do not increase significantly until the second and third trimesters, when the majority of fetal growth occurs and most of the additional nutrients are needed (Ritchie and King 2008). While energy requirements of pregnant women vary depending on the mother's basal metabolic rate, pregravid weight, weight gain during pregnancy, activity levels, and state of pregnancy, on average, women don't need more than 300 extra daily calories during their second and third trimesters to meet their nutritional needs during the prenatal period (Ritchie and King 2008). Additionally, these calories (and others) should be provided by nutrient-rich foods (as opposed to calorie-dense, low nutrient foods) (Ritchie and King 2008). Excessive weight gain during pregnancy or overnutrition can lead to a variety of poor health outcomes, including gestational diabetes, macrosomia, possible complications with delivery, and can lead to increased propensity for overweight and obesity in offspring (Ritchie and King 2008). Undernutrition can also lead to health complications, such as low birth weight and intrauterine growth retardation. Both low birth weight and macrosomia have been linked with increased risk for chronic disease in offspring (e.g., hypertension, cardiovascular disease, type 2 diabetes, and metabolic syndrome) (Godfrey 2006).

Beyond energy requirements there are increased requirements for specific macronutrients (i.e., proteins, fats, and carbohydrates) and micronutrients (i.e., vitamins and minerals). For example, requirements for proteins[2] increase since they help with fetal growth, placental development, amniotic fluid, maternal blood volume, and regulation of other maternal tissues (Ritchie and King 2008). The requirements for some water-soluble vitamins, such as folate[3] and vitamin B6, substantially increase through the course of the pregnancy (Ritchie and King 2008), as folate deficiency is associated with neural tube defects, which occur in the weeks following conception, making it imperative that women consume foods fortified with folic acid and dietary supplements in the preconception period. Vitamin B6 is involved with various metabolic reactions and is associated with improved pregnancy outcomes (i.e., reduced preeclampsia and higher Apgar scores) (Ritchie and King 2008). Some minerals, such as iron are also important during pregnancy. Maternal iron-deficiency[4] anemia is the most common nutrition-related pregnancy complication, but iron deficiency in the fetus and newborns is rare since the neonate will draw on the mother's hepatic iron stores (Ritchie and King 2008). Although requirements for other nutrients, such as calcium, do not increase, it is still important to have adequate nutrient intake to avoid pregnancy complications, which can lead to health problems for the mother and child. There are additional dietary recommendations agreed upon by experts, such as lowering caffeine intake to less than 200 milligrams daily (e.g., a 12 oz. cup of coffee), limiting intake of seafood that contains mercury (e.g., white albacore tuna), maintaining proper food handling to avoid food poisoning (e.g., washing fruits and vegetables and cooking meats properly), and avoiding listeriosis (Montero et al. 2015) by eliminating consumption of unpasteurized dairy products, smoked seafood, and lunch meats[5] (ACOG 2018).

The literature on the nutrition transition outlines various characteristics that define this phenomenon. This includes high fat intake, added sugars, refined carbohydrates, and animal-source foods (Popkin 2015).

High Fat Intake and Animal-source Foods

There was a link between high fat intake and animal-source foods, as all the contributors to high saturated fat intake for pregnant women were animal-source foods. There was a higher than recommended intake of saturated fats across the sample overall, especially during the second and third trimester (26.81 grams vs. <20 grams) (n=21), but also for a couple of women who were in their first trimester (23.45 grams vs. 20 grams). While research indicates that women should limit their intake of saturated fats during pregnancy due to the risk for gestational diabetes (Shin et al. 2015), all women in this sample had normal blood sugar at the time of the interview. It is possible that women in their earlier trimesters developed high blood glucose later on in their pregnancy, but I did not have access to this information. Pregnant women did not report any negative health effects that could be linked to high saturated fat intake, although it is also possible there were other items in the diet that are buffering women from the negative effects of high saturated fat intake.

Animal-source foods were associated with cravings for processed meats, price, avoiding processed meats, and *chatarra*. Some pregnant women talked about their food cravings for processed meats, which included hamburgers, sliced sandwich meat, and sausage. One participant noted that she ate these types of foods because they were cheaper. Others noted that consumption of these meats has increased due to lack of time today to prepare other foods. It is easier to eat the premade ready meats with work and school schedules. However, there was also consensus that some animal-source foods should be avoided due to health reasons. Women talked about avoiding some traditional meat products, such as fried pork rinds, due to the high amount of lard used for cooking. This was particularly difficult for some participants who admitted that their husbands often want this typical dish, as well as other meat dishes. As one older woman noted, "My husband is addicted to pork, so now we have eliminated almost all meat" (Alma, 41). For women in the sample, the idea of street food and fast foods, like hamburgers, fried chicken, and pizza, was lumped into the category of "junk foods." This also included fried meats and hamburgers. There was recognition that these foods have a high percentage of fat and that's why they should be avoided. One woman noted that she used to only eat hamburgers when she left the Monteverde Zone and now many places in town serve hamburgers, including a fast food kiosk on the main street.

Based on my previous research in the region, I hypothesized that the high saturated fat intake would be attributed to junk foods, such as pizza or hamburgers. However, the majority of foods that contributed to fat intake were items that make up the local culinary tradition in the area. This includes, farmer's cheese, sausage, chicken soup, and beef stew. As this is a historically agricultural region, which has relied on dairy farming and used to have two pig farms which sold their meat to the cheese factory for sausage, these items are typical.

Added Sugars and Refined Carbohydrates

Although the nutritional data do not reflect an excess intake of sugars or refined carbohydrates within the sample overall, some participants did consumed sweetened iced teas (n=2) and Tang (n=2). Some also consumed packaged and processed foods, such as packaged cookies (n=3), crackers (n=1), chips (n=2), caramel popcorn (n=1), and skittles (n=1). As these results show, the intake of these items was low within the sample.

There were some notable micronutrient deficiencies, such as vitamin D, vitamin A, iron, potassium, and alpha tocopherol. However, all women in the sample were taking prenatal vitamins, which would make up for the deficits in the dietary sources of the micronutrients. Although previous research has shown that this region is experiencing a tourism-driven nutrition transition, pregnant women appeared to be adhering to prescribed dietary practices and cultural beliefs which promoted healthy diets overall.

Dietary Delocalization

Dietary delocalization is also a key feature of the nutrition transition and can be tied to tourism-development in the region. While diets consisted mostly of local and traditional food items, such as rice, beans, and fruit, typical dishes were delocalized in terms of their ingredients. The replacement of natural ingredients with packaged and processed foods, such as packaged meats (in place of locally produced meats) and powdered dairy products (in place of locally produced milk), can lead to negative impacts on health. For example, the World Health Organization recently announced that processed meats are categorized as carcinogenic (i.e., cancer causing) (WHO 2016).

Dietary delocalization can occur via many pathways. Tourism-related infrastructure is perhaps the most direct avenue of change for this community. As a direct result of pressure from the tourism industry, the communities in the Monteverde Zone voted to pave the road from the Pan-American Highway up to Monteverde. Construction began in 2014 and continues to date. The road has been a contentious issue for locals, as many believe that the road will bring too many tourists. Further, some corruption regarding funds has resulted in a half-finished project, which in many places has left the road in worse conditions than when they started. Not only do better quality roads signify that more tourists will have access to the Monteverde Zone but it also means that different nonlocal food products are coming into the region. Participants talked about the desire for some of these food items due to their increased access (e.g., the availability of pizza makes people want pizza). Although there was always a supermarket in Monteverde in recent history, today there are two new major chains that have stores throughout Latin America and the Caribbean, along with a locally owned store and numerous smaller mini-mart–type shops called *pulperías*. One participant commented that when there were no supermarkets, there were no chips and no sodas. There is also the thought that people in Monteverde Zone want to be more modern and can do this through the consumption of purchased food items (i.e., cornflakes and boxed milk). This was reflected by the food cravings described by pregnant women, for foods such as pizza, hamburgers, Nutella, and kiwis, which are not produced locally. Some pregnant women also indicated that the prices of foods are high because everything comes from outside of the region. As one pregnant woman said, "Foods that come from outside of the zone, those, yes, are a little bit more. For example, if you want to eat *ceviche* or something that has fish, it's going to be more expensive here because everything is brought here from outside of the zone, so it's going to be more expensive" (Estela, 25, 4 months pregnant). Estela went on to say, "Almost everything [is more expensive], yes, because everything comes from outside of the zone, so even the rice is more expensive."

Health

Despite evidence showing links between the nutrition transition and risk for adverse health outcomes in rural community, pregnant women who participated in this study had adequate nutrition and did not seem to be affected by the negative health impacts commonly associated with the nutrition transition. Health among pregnant women was good overall. All pregnant women (n=22) had blood pressure within a normal range. Women also reported having blood sugar within a normal range and birth weight and gestational age for those who were available for a follow-up conversation were normal. I also collected height and pregravid weight as biological markers of nutrition in order to calculate pregravid body mass index, which was, on average, 25.32. This placed women, on average, in the overweight body mass index category. While this could be a factor for health risks during pregnancy, women did not report any health problems during their pregnancies. Even though research shows that this community is impacted by tourism-driven nutrition transition, pregnant women seem to be buffered from the negative health effects by a strong sense of shared cultural identity which encourages them to engage in locally defined prenatal dietary practices.

NOTES

1. Twenty-four-hour diet recall data were imported into Diet Analysis Plus software (Wadsworth 2011) for nutritional assessment. Some food equivalents were not available within the software program. In these cases, research was conducted using the USDA Food Tracker (USDA 2015) in order to find a suitable equivalent that was in the Diet Analysis Plus database. Notes were recorded in the Excel database file to indicate when foods were replaced with food equivalents in analysis.

2. The protein requirement during gestation is 71 grams per day (Institute of Medicine 2011).

3. The current dietary recommended intake for folic acid is 600 micrograms daily (from both dietary sources and supplements) (ACOG 2018).

4. It is recommended that women consume 27 milligrams of iron daily, which can usually be provided by dietary supplements (ACOG 2018).

5. Although this is not a comprehensive review of macro and micronutrient requirements during pregnancy, the nutrients listed are the most relevant to this investigation and were chosen due to their importance during gestation.

Chapter 7

Engaging in Practice

Decision-Making and Human Agency

The center of town had changed a lot since my first visit in 2008. While some landmarks remained the same, such as the Catholic Church and the local bar, tourism had become a more prominent feature of this once rural community. At the time the research for this book was conducted, there was a large digital billboard in the small downtown plaza that constantly ran ads for local adventure tourism, mostly zip lines and rappelling. There were also a lot more food options, ranging from fast food kiosks, which sold items such as fried chicken, hamburgers, and French fries, to finer dining establishments with tablecloths and cloth napkins. On one particular day I was headed into the latter to interview a young woman who worked for her family-owned business. I arrived in the mid-morning and the restaurant was empty, but I could hear the clanking of silverware and plates in the back. A woman in her forties with dark hair and a chef's coat came out to greet me. Lisa's mother was the owner of the restaurant and the chef. I introduced myself and we chatted for a few minutes before Lisa showed up. The wide smile on her face extended into her crystal clear blue eyes. Lisa was already 7.5 months pregnant when I interviewed her and the excitement about meeting her new son was apparent. She explained to me that she and her boyfriend both worked at her family's restaurant full time. This interview was different than many others. First, the setting of a modern and upscale restaurant in the center of town was a contrast to the other places I conducted interviews: in women's modest homes made of crudely painted wood or concrete, or in public spaces of convenience for participants. Second, the fact that the restaurant had a female owner and chef was somewhat unique. While female business owners were more common in the zone, this still did not reflect the dominant gender norms, where men were the heads of the household. Because of these two characteristics, I presumed that this interview would be different than the others and that Lisa's responses to questions about localized cultural practices may differ from those of my other participants who seemed to share more socioeconomic characteristics. I was completely wrong. The shared beliefs about prenatal diet were common across the sample. For example, Lisa described an experience she had eating spicy peppers and linked this directly with shared cultural beliefs about pregnancy.

Lisa: Yes, at first I got an obsession with chili peppers, I added chili peppers to everything. And in fact, in this Mexican restaurant my husband bought me two orders of jalapeño peppers and I ate them. My mom told me not to because of the baby. I don't know if he [the baby] knew it was coming or what, but he started to move and move and I don't know if it was because he was upset. I don't really know. But I stopped completely [eating chili peppers] because if he had that reaction that he was moving and moving and I don't know if it was the chili peppers.

ME: Ok, but that was more because of the baby's reaction, not because someone told you not to eat chili peppers?

Lisa: Yes, they told me that since that [the chili peppers] were going into the amniotic fluid, then the baby was going to be born burned.

ME: The skin?

Lisa: Yes.

Lisa contextualized her experience with the belief that spicy food could result in the baby being born *piel manchada*, or with hives or red splotches. This fit within a broader narrative that women told about wanting their babies to be born with clean skin. Overall, there were shared ideas about cultural beliefs that guided prenatal decision-making regarding diet. Various cultural beliefs, or *creencias*, emerged through participant interviews (n=42), identifying the ways in which culture influences decision-making about prenatal dietary behaviors. In addition to cultural beliefs, other constructs surfaced as the most prevalent trends while exploring food-related decision-making among women, including knowledge, social actors, and food access. There is also evidence to suggest that the process of decision-making surrounding prenatal dietary practices has shifted over time. This information is key in understanding trends in community health related to the tourism-driven nutrition transition.

CONSTRUCTS OF HUMAN AGENCY

While my emphasis on an agency-oriented approach diverges from Ortner's work, her focus on social interactions with the idea of serious games is central to the analysis presented here. Four agency-oriented constructs were applied in this context, including: "intentionality," "negotiation," "reproduction," and "resistance" (Ortner 1997). These constructs were drawn from Ortner's (1997) juxtaposition of the construction of subjects and the making of subjects, and they were analyzed in relation to the influence of other social actors, building the bridge between "individual" agency and Ortner's (1997) idea that agency is not individual, but is embedded in social interactions and relationships from which it cannot be removed. I will describe the methodology here in order to highlight the unique contribution that this application of practice theory makes. This model is not only useful for subdisciplinary theory building, but also expands how we can think about health, by taking into account various aspects of human decision-making in a systematic, reproducible way. Other studies have used practice theory to understand dietary practices, such as snacking (Twine 2015; Weijzen et al. 2009), food and eating as social practice (Southerton 2012; Delormier et al. 2009), and children's food practices (Punch et al. 2010). However, the way that data was synthesized for this book is unique.

In applying Ortner's construction of human agency (1997) to pregnant women's experiences with decision-making in the Monteverde Zone, "intentionality" (n=38) was identified in women's narrative if they discussed specific dietary behaviors in a way that suggested premeditated thought about a decision they had made in the past (in the case of women with older children), or indicated that they had a plan to engage in specific dietary practices in the future (in the case of pregnant women) (e.g., plan to drink flaxseed a few weeks before their due date). In some instances a clear "negotiation" (n=41) was present in the narrative, characterized by the uncertainty expressed by the participant regarding decisions about prenatal dietary practices (e.g., when women discussed the factors that influenced their decision on where to purchase food, such as food prices). These sections of text were identified as, negotiation. Further, these intentions and negotiations involved the "reproduction" (n=39) of culturally appropriate dietary practices (i.e., foods for benefits, food taboos, food avoidances, and food cravings) where the participant engages in the same practices that are part of the cultural milieu (e.g., following the taboo not to eat spicy foods). "Resistance" (n=29) occurred when the participant indicated that they did not or would not participate in specific dietary practices, or if they indicated that they did not want to participate in a typical practice (e.g., when referring to the taboo against drinking certain teas as a "myth" and indicating that they weren't going follow that practice).

These four conceptual categories were analyzed in relation to one another, and in relation to four constructs in the context of prenatal dietary practices using a code co-occurrence analysis. Atlas.ti (2013), a qualitative analysis software, has a function that allows the user to examine the ways in which coded segments of text overlap and to explore the relationship between concepts (Namey et al. 2008). A code co-occurrence is present if one quotation is coded with two codes. The code co-occurrence table identifies the frequency with which two codes overlap. Additionally, code co-occurrences are analyzed as part of a matrix (similar to a correlation matrix in statistics) and a c-coefficient is produced. This number ranges from 0 to 1 and reflects the strength of the relationship between the two codes. This is similar to a correlation coefficient, with 0 being no relationship and 1 being a very strong relationship. This is a preliminary tool that is best used with larger sample sizes (greater than twenty). By examining the relationship between cultural beliefs, knowledge, social actors, and food access, with dimensions of human agency, I unpack the decision-making processes involved with prenatal dietary behavior. I also compare pregnant women's experiences with those of older women in order to better assess how decision-making has changed over time in the context of tourism development and shifting foodways associated with the nutrition transition.

CULTURAL BELIEFS

Cultural beliefs mentioned in the previous chapter (*boca abierta*, hot foods, an emphasis on clean skin, and the belief that some teas could cause miscarriages or spontaneous abortions) were not associated with constructs of human agency for pregnant women. In contrast, cultural beliefs overlapped with all constructs of human agency for older women. The strongest relationships occurred with the reproduction (n=14, c-coefficient=.11) and resistance (n=8, c-coefficient=.16) to practices. In other words, older women talked about reproducing dietary practices associated with cultural beliefs or resisting them. One woman explained why she drank flaxseed after seven or eight months of her pregnancy, and she said, "And for me, I like to drink it because my grandmother, my grandmother would say to drink flaxseed so that my kids would have clean skin. So, I don't know if it's true, but my kids have perfect skin" (Alma, 41). This particular sentiment is juxtaposed with the belief that flaxseed is taboo earlier in pregnancy. Interestingly, there is some evidence to suggest that there is an association between consumption of flaxseed and increased risk of preterm birth (Moussally and Bérard 2010). This is relevant to the data presented here, as women commonly consumed flaxseed with water as their due dates approached, but identified it as a taboo item to consume earlier in pregnancy. The belief is that this will help the baby to come quicker and to make the overall birth process smoother.

Among dietary practices for pregnant women, food taboos (n=10, c-coefficient=.26) showed the strongest relationship with cultural beliefs, meaning women were adhering to food taboos in the context of these belief systems. Dietary taboos included restricting intake of certain foods because of beliefs about hot/cold disease theory, items that cause abortion or miscarriage, and items that can affect the cleanliness of the newborn's skin. These same constructs are common in the cross-cultural literature among various cultural groups in Africa, Iran, India, and Malaysia (Arzoaquoi et al. 2015; Phillips 2005; Ahlqvist and Wirfalt 2000; Choudry 1997; Laderman 1987). Among older women, results were similar as food taboos had the highest degree of association with the cultural beliefs. These findings reflect the degree of the relationship between cultural beliefs identified by participants and their prenatal dietary practices. This fits with the data that show that "hot" foods, such as teas and spicy items, were considered taboo during pregnancy, and in practice, women did not consume these items. Items that were considered too "hot" and could cause an abortion or miscarriage included teas, such as chamomile and rosemary. While most commercially produced teas are safe to consume during pregnancy (American Pregnancy Association 2016), problems can arise when teas contain excessive amounts of herbs or are made with toxic substances. Two separate Italian studies found that regular consumption of chamomile (i.e., daily consumption) during pregnancy was statistically linked with lower birth weight (Trabace et al. 2015; Facchinetti et al. 2012). Johns and Sibeko (2003) note that oxytoxic and uterine-stimulating herbs such as chamomiles, parsley, rosemary, and rue could cause spontaneous abortion. However, this is dependent on dosage. Additionally, some chamomiles, such as German and Russian chamomiles, could also be problematic during pregnancy due to properties that can make them potential allergens (Johns and Sibeko 2003). However, another study found no increased risk for prematurity among women who consumed chamomile, peppermint, or green tea in the last two trimesters of pregnancy (Moussally and Bérard 2010). While non-herbal teas, such as green tea, have antioxidants, these teas also contain caffeine. Other foods that were considered "hot" were avoided (e.g., hot peppers) because they could "burn" their baby's skin, resulting in hives. The belief that consuming hot foods during pregnancy can cause hives in newborns has been noted in other regions of Latin America, such as Argentina (Martínez 2008). Interestingly, some women also believed that Coca-Cola could cause the same reaction. While there is no evidence to suggest that this is true, this is one way that women have adapted to the new food environments. In this case, the local belief about newborn's clean skin is adaptive in that it may buffer women from the negative effects of drinking too much soda (i.e., high sugar intake associated with the nutrition transition).

Based on these findings, cultural beliefs may play a similar role in influencing dietary practices among pregnant women today and older women (who were pregnant over fifteen years ago). However, these results also show that cultural beliefs may not have as much influence over different constructs of human agency as they did in the past. This distinction is important. While women are still adhering to some practices associated with cultural beliefs, the process by which this is occurring is changing. There may be other driving forces today that influence the ways that women make decisions regarding prenatal diet. It's relevant for health promotion to understand these new pathways involved with decision-making.

FOOD ACCESS

Food access emerged a conceptual grouping that included cost, growing season, source, and tourism season. Two aspects of food access, cost (n=16) and food sources (n=38), were associated with the negotiation (n=15, c-coefficient=.13) (n=10, c-coefficient=.07) that pregnant women went through when making decisions about dietary practices. This is not surprising, as economic factors were also mentioned by free listing respondents as something that influences nutrition in the Monteverde Zone. As one pregnant woman explained, "Ok, sometimes it is a little bit difficult because you want to buy a lot of things, a lot of fruits, or something healthy, and sometimes, therefore, economically, you can't" (Ines, 22, 8 months pregnant). Although all women recognized that they needed to eat a healthy diet during their pregnancy, they were faced with the high food costs associated with life in the Monteverde Zone. Just as women had to be strategic about how they could eat healthy during their pregnancies, they also took the food source into consideration. Food in the region came from various sources: (1) supermarket in town (one of three), (2) supermarket outside of town, (3) *pulpería* (small corner stores with minimal fresh foods), (4) home garden, (5) food sharing, (6) mobile vendors (men on motorcycles that sold vegetables, fish, or baked goods), and (7) local farmers who sold their products directly. The decision about where to obtain food was influenced by the cost of food, the cost of transportation, and the needs of the household. In some cases, as in the example presented earlier, some women's families or neighbors grew food or had cows, which provided at least some household items throughout the year. Another pregnant woman (Estela, 25, 4.5 months pregnant) lived close to her in-laws, and while she grows some basic ingredients at her house (e.g., cilantro), she often eats at her in-laws on the weekends. Further, they have cows so they give them milk and cheese products, and they provide them with large chunks of natural salt. This family also buys beans from a local farmer in bulk so they have enough throughout the year. However, the relationship with her in-laws can be tough sometimes. As Estela notes, it's the influence of the family that encourages her to eat larger portions while she is pregnant, although she has struggled with being overweight during her pregnancy and knows that she shouldn't overeat. She said,

> Yes, because it is a little bit difficult with them [in-laws] because they want to give you food all the time, right? And more during pregnancy, saying you have to eat more. But, regardless, I made the decision not to, I can't take it anymore, no, no, no I am not going to eat it. "No thank you, I am not going to eat it." Or I serve myself a little bit. If I already know that there is food prepared, then I'm going to eat just a little bit, right? So that I don't get that full. Because I am going to eat the ration I always eat, but then they bring me more and I'm not going to be able to eat it. So, if it's a situation like that, where I already know there is food prepared, I am going to eat a little bit, right, so that I can eat a little more when they bring more. (Estela, 25, 4.5 months pregnant)

Similar to pregnant women, there was an association between negotiation and food source (n=8, c-coefficient=.05) that took place for older women when they were pregnant in the Monteverde Zone, although cost was not a factor tied in with human agency. These findings suggest that cost is an emerging characteristic of the food environment which bears on decision-making and supports other findings presented in this book, such as the emphasis placed on economic factors by free listing participants when asked about influences on nutrition in the region. However, as one participant noted, there were less options. She said,

> Before there was a very small corner store and only the traders would take all the best, all the best vegetables. And we would go and we would have to buy what remained, what people left. Let's say, second-class fruit, like the potato, everything that was the best quality they took, like onion, cucumber, everything. So we would arrive on the 15th of the month, then we would buy what others left, because we didn't have another way to get to Puntarenas. It already cost a lot to go to Puntarenas. To go to Tilarán also, so we would have to buy everything there, in that same store, here. But not now, *mami*. Now there is Mega Super and the other grocery store and the farmer's market. Before there wasn't a farmer's market. There wasn't a farmer's market. Now there is the farmer's market, the grocery store and it's much easier to buy things. (Angelica 44)

Additionally, it was much harder for women to travel around the Monteverde Zone (and in and out of the zone). As one older woman said,

> But it was very difficult to go to Santa Elena where they sold a lot of the fruits. It was difficult to eat fruits during that time. If you didn't go to Santa Elena you couldn't eat many fruits. The corner store was further from here and they didn't have many fruits. Sometimes they did, but normally they didn't. So the fruits that I ate were from Santa Elena, but it was difficult to get there without

> transportation because it was very expensive. With my first pregnancy we didn't have electricity, so we only bought a little bit to keep because we didn't have a refrigerator. It was very difficult. (Melissa, 51)

This participant's oldest child was twenty-nine years old, reflecting the rapid changes that have occurred in the region over the last thirty years or so. During the time that this woman spoke of there was no paved road leading to this particular community and no electricity. Today, the road is paved and is travelled daily by taxis and school buses. This also makes access easier for the mobile vendors. Older women also indicated that they received most of their food from farms (either their own or others). One woman noted, "I think, I think from the farm, yes. I think we also got food from the farm. My husband has always liked to grow food, so we always had a lot, yes. Like vegetables, a lot of vegetables. Like yucca, green beans, and oranges. And if there wasn't anything up here, in the lower neighborhoods we had friends that had something. After that, plantains, bananas, and sweet potato too" (Emma, 51). Another older woman shared that sentiment and said,

> Yes, before we did a lot of that. For example, here with our friends we could exchange a lot. They had a lot of spinach, we would exchange for bananas. We would take something, and they would take something else. We did that more before, yes, a lot before. Now, no, it's less. Yes, sometimes there is a neighbor who says, "I have a lot of this, do you want some?" Or like we have bananas here, so we will call our neighbors, "do you want bananas?" There are a lot of *maduro* bananas. They get exchanged. Even though more people grew food, they still bought some staples. We almost always bought some things. We had everything on the farm. We bought rice, oil and salt. We had to go to Santa Elena or Las Juntas on horseback to bring those items back. (Samantha, 60)

For pregnant women and older women constructs associated with food access (cost, growing season, source, and tourism season) were not relevant to any prenatal dietary practices, indicating that cost and food source are influential factors when it comes to food-related behaviors in general, but not specifically for prenatal dietary practices. It is possible that pregnancy provides a buffer to these access issues, although these data do not speak directly to this hypothesis.

KNOWLEDGE

Knowledge emerged as another trend in the data and included previous pregnancy experience (n=7), previous experience with prenatal care (n=4), and sources of information. For pregnant women, there was a relationship between information from the family (n=21) and negotiation (n=17, c-coefficient=.08) and reproduction (n=15, c-coefficient=.08) of dietary practices. There was also a relationship between information from the clinic (n=22) and the reproduction (n= 8, c-coefficient= .07) of dietary practices. Overall, pregnant women received information about prenatal diet from various sources, including: family, the clinic, private doctor, school, friends, the Internet, television, books, magazines, and phone applications. When asked about where they received the most information about prenatal dietary practices, pregnant women indicated that it came from the clinic (n=6). While some pregnant women said the most information came from their families (n=5), an equal number of women said they didn't receive any information from any source (n=5). Four women indicated that the majority of information came from a mixed source (a mixture of family, friends, the clinic, private care, and/or the Internet) and two pregnant women said they received the majority of information from the Internet.

Two structural entities were most associated with decision-making: the family and the clinic. As one participant noted, "You always try to do what they say. The parents in your family maybe because of their experience, because they are older and they know more. And, in the clinic because the doctors always tell you what's best" (Rebecca, 18, 7 months pregnant). It is possible that information from other sources influenced women's agency and decision-making, but it was not reflected in their narrative about prenatal dietary practices. Information from the family was associated with negotiation and reproduction of prenatal dietary practices. Information that came from the clinic was also associated with the reproduction of practices, but not with negotiation. There was more overlap in the narrative of instances where women reproduced practices in the context of advice from family than the clinic (15. vs. 8, respectively), although the strength of the relationship was similar, However, the fact that information from the clinic is associated with the reproduction of dietary practices also reflects the status of the clinic and biomedical knowledge in decision-making in this context.

Families provided information about prenatal supplements, foods that have dietary benefits (e.g., fruits), foods to avoid (e.g., foods with a lot of fat), and diet taboos (e.g., spicy foods). Family members also encouraged pregnant women to stop eating junk foods, such as bags of chips, sodas, and fast foods. In many cases, pregnant women negotiated the information that they received from their family. For example, the woman described in this chapter's introduction didn't heed her mother's advice about consuming hot peppers, but after her own experience decided to follow this food taboo. In this case, her experiential knowledge played a role in reinforcing this cultural norms. Another woman explained how her family gave her advice about her cravings. "If you are craving something, 'then eat,' if you have a heavy desire to eat, 'then eat.'" She went on to explain, "That's because they say that after the baby comes, I don't know, the baby will come out with cravings or will barely eat so, so that's so the baby is also okay. So, let's say, if I want to eat a lot of chocolate, I need to eat it because the baby wants it, but I also know that it is not good to eat that much, so maybe I'll just eat a little bit" (Marina, 25, 6 months pregnant). Family also played a more materialistic role (i.e., providing material food items, not just information) in the reproduction of dietary practices of pregnant women. In some cases women explained that they ate what their mothers or mothers-in-law made for them, or the foods that their family provided for them. For example, one woman said,

> My father is someone who is always growing food. so, even if there isn't something prepared, of some food, he is going to have something because he is always cultivating food. So this is an easy option because he always has yucca, sweet potato, plantains, bananas, squashes, and in general he always grows a lot of cilantro. So maybe in other places there isn't the option but here you can eat what grows in the farm. Or, he comes with a lot of food and says, "take this for yourself," and that is an option that is very easy and you don't have to buy something. (Rebecca, 19, 8 months pregnant)

This leads to the reproduction of local dietary behaviors, as the foods grown on the farm are part of the food culture of this region. Food sharing of local fruits also helps with the reproduction of this practice and to enforce the advice from family and the clinic that pregnant women should eat fruits during their pregnancy because of their benefits.

Information that women received from the clinic was also associated with reproduction of dietary practices, although there was variation in women's narrative on decision-making. Women agreed that they didn't have much time with the doctor during their monthly prenatal exams, although they did receive information during their short visit. The recommendations were to eat fruits, vegetables, and beans, and to avoid salt and sugars. The doctors also stressed the importance of taking prenatal vitamins (folic acid and iron), which were provided for free. Additionally, clinic staff provided medical explanations for some food taboos that pregnant women heard from their families. As one pregnant woman said, "In the clinic they say that since chamomile, young coconut water, and honey are anti-inflammatories, they are used a lot when someone has a bad stomach and so if you drink these things during your pregnancy your body will treat the baby as an infection, or something bad and will try and get rid of it" (Rebecca, 21, 8.5 months pregnant). Some women agreed that they don't really receive a lot of nutritional information from the clinic, but that they can ask the nurse or doctor about practices that their families have shared with them. As one pregnant woman said, "No, I, well, in reality it's more like one of those days I asked, 'is it true that flaxseed is bad to drink during pregnancy?' They said, 'yes, it's bad.' So, um, ok. But in reality they don't give much information about specific foods or anything like that" (Jordana, 22, 5.5 months pregnant). One pregnant woman explained that the information from the clinic doesn't impact her decisions. She said, "No, because in the clinic they are simply going to tell you the same thing, to continue eating the same amounts of food, that you shouldn't eat too much just because you are pregnant and that you should eat more fruits and vegetables. It's practically all the advice they give you, right? And drink a lot of liquids, right, enough water, things like that. But, it's not like very detailed, right?" (Estela, 25, 4.5 months pregnant). Another pregnant woman agreed, "Very, very basic, like there was a lack of information. More than anything it's what I look for on the internet." She went on to say, "It was very basic. 'Try and eat more fruit, drink a lot of liquids, oatmeal.' Things with yogurt for example, in my case because I was a bit constipated. Cereals with fiber. And nothing else" (Jessica, 34, 8 months pregnant).

In contrast, some women explained that they received detailed information from the clinic. For example, one of these pregnant women said,

> No, well they recommended eating more salads. Yes, with lettuce. Eating more red meat and liver, because it has a lot of iron. They recommended eating eggs because they have a lot of protein. Milk for the calcium. I don't know, with each meal that I make I have to eat a snack an hour or hour and half later, after my meal. A fruit, or something that has proteins. Drink a lot of liquids, a lot of water, when you are already pregnant you are susceptible to more infections and miscarriage, so you should drink a lot of water. Take care of yourself, don't do heavy exercise, and walk, for moderate amounts of time, not too much because this can dilate your hips and the baby can come. Okay, well, that's what they told me at the clinic, right, the times I went and they gave me information. (María, 18, 6 months pregnant)

Similarly, the clinic and family members were the main sources of information discussed in older women's narratives. The clinic (n=19) was associated with the reproduction (n=9, c-coefficient=.05) of practices, as was the family (n=16) (n=10, c-coefficient=.07). The family was also associated with negotiation (n=8, c-coefficient=.06) of dietary practices. Most of the women with older children did have access to healthcare, as the clinic in Santa Elena originally opened in the 1970s, although the health post in the neighboring community was not yet established. One older woman also indicated that they got basic advice from the clinic during their pregnancies. She said, "Like more than anything how to take care of myself. What do I know? They say that it was good to eat fruit and foods with iron during pregnancy. Yes, that was the most they explained to me" (Emma, 51). Similarly to many pregnant women, one older woman explained that she didn't receive information about nutrition from the clinic during her visits. She said, "Not that type of information, no. It is like a normal appointment. They are going to measure your stomach, listen to the heartbeat, but no, no. They don't tell you anything during the appointment about what you should eat, no nothing like that" (Isabella, 34). Isabella went on to say, "During that time, really, you didn't receive that much information. Basically when you went to your control visit in the clinic. They would make some comments, but it wasn't a lot of information in that time." Another older woman explained the degree to which things have changed. She explained that one of her relatives gave her a book about pregnancy. She said,

> Yes, and it said everything that would happen, like when you are going to have a baby. It told you what to do and what not to do. But in that time it was prohibited to have those books. In that time all of that was prohibited by the family. You couldn't even realize, right, how you were going to have a child. Unless you got information from doctors or mothers, but I remember that my mother never fully explained those things to me, because she barely knew herself. What to do, right? She had her kids but there were a lot of things that she didn't know, right? And so I had my first daughter at age 21. I had my daughter. But, everything went well. I had my births, and everything went well. (Julia, 61)

Since women didn't have access to the Internet or smartphones at that time, some would get little pamphlets or books when they could. From family, women with older children received similar advice. One woman noted, "Yes, from the family I was practicing with what my mother would eat, or what my mother would say: 'okay, eat more chicken soup, more vegetables, yes, and don't eat too many sweets'" (Alba). Family also gave advice about specific foods that helped with anemia, such as a specific type of cilantro (i.e., *culantro coyote*) that was to be mixed in with beans and a plantain-like fruit (i.e., *guineo negro*) that is rich in iron.

The respective overlaps between the clinic and the family, the negotiation and reproduction of dietary practices for pregnant women was most relevant when it came to dietary taboos and foods consumed for benefits. For older women, this was similar, although these sources of information were most influential when it came to benefits (family and clinic) and avoidances (clinic). These results indicate that these sources of information may have remained stable over time, which may also account for the stability in adherence to food taboos, as family members would pass down this information.

SOCIAL ACTORS

Social actors emerged as a trend in the data, as individuals in the lives of participants seem to influence constructs of human agency and dietary decision-making. Additionally, due to Ortner's (2006) emphasis on the construction of human agency as embedded in social contexts, this construct fits well with the theoretical underpinnings of the analysis. This conceptual grouping included sixteen social actors for pregnant women and twenty-four for women with older children (see table 7.1). All social actors were identified if they were discussed in the context of prenatal dietary practices or food-related decision-making.

Overall, twenty-four social actors were discussed by women in the study. However, only sixteen social actors were part of pregnant women's narrative, including: sister-in-law, doctor, father, grandparents, kids, mother, neighbors, nurses, parents, siblings, private doctor, friends, partner, mother-in-law, father-in-law, and aunt. The social actors discussed by the most pregnant women were mothers, partners, friends, mothers-in-law, and nurses.

The only social actors who were influential in shaping human agency among pregnant women were mothers-in-law. Mothers-in-law were associated with negotiation (n=6, c-coefficient=.05) and reproduction (n=4, c-coefficient=.05) of dietary taboos. In some cases women were reliant on their mothers-in-law for support during their pregnancies since their own mothers lived outside of the Monteverde Zone. For the most part women viewed this as helpful. One woman who moved to the Monteverde Zone from the Central Valley said, "My mother-in-law, she is my right hand" (Caroline, 24, 6.5 months pregnant). Another pregnant woman noted, "She [her mother-in-law] helps me a lot with nutrition because she tries to give me a lot of healthy foods, buy me fruits, milk, and yogurt" (Rebecca, 21, 8.5 months pregnant). During this interview this participant's mother-in-law was present and agreed that she tried to prepare healthy meals for her to eat. "I bring steak, I bring her chicken, and I make a sauce. Steak or chicken breast. Things like that and nothing else. And sometimes I make a squash hash dish because my daughter likes it. I make it for her [the pregnant woman], but I don't think she likes it very much, right?" Rebecca responded hesitantly, "Well, more or less. It depends. It depends on the type of hash." Her mother-in-law responded happily, "So, that's what I give her." This narrative reflects the ways that mothers-in-law have the power to influence what their daughters-in-law eat, especially when they live together. In this example, Rebecca indicated that she only liked hash dishes (which are very typical of this area) if they were prepared in a certain way. The mother-in-law's tone in this situation reflected her pride in the fact that she could provide this healthy dish to her family. However, not every narrative reflected the same amicability as this one. In another example, one pregnant woman was asked to reflect on her own nutrition. She said, "Well, my nutrition is good, it's not bad" (María, 18, 6 months pregnant). However, her mother-in-law immediately chimed in and said, "But in general when you are pregnant you have anemia, you need a lot more iron. And that is what I was telling

Table 7.1 Social Actors and Decision-Making

Social Actors	*Pregnant Women* *N*	*Women with Older Children* *N*
Sister-in-Law	1	4
Brother-in-Law	X	3
Clinic Doctor	6	16
Employer	X	2
Father	3	9
Grandparents	3	10
Kids	6	X
Mother	16	18
Neighbors	2	4
Nurses	9	8
Parents	2	1
Midwife	X	5
Siblings	7	9
Private Doctor	6	6
Friends	10	11
Partner	18	17
Mother-in-Law	9	9
Father-in-Law	2	2
Aunt	1	4

her, because she is working and she goes without lunch, without dinner. When you don't have a [pregnant] belly you can endure hunger all day if you want. But with a [pregnant] belly or when you are breastfeeding, never. She has to pull something out, whether it is fruit, or a sandwich, she has to bring something to pull through the afternoon, she has to eat something in the afternoon. And she has to, I always tell her, 'breakfast will be ready, lunch will be ready,' because we make lunch at the house, but she should get dinner ready and take a sandwich, with cheese and tomato, or however, she wants." María responded, "Well, I always bring a snack." Her mother-in-law said, "But you can't go hungry and that is one of the things that you are doing. She doesn't want to eat in the afternoon because there is nowhere to heat up the food. It doesn't matter if it's cold, eat it." María continued, "Well, yes, I frequently eat fruit. Yes, I eat fruits and I bring my snack, yes." In contrast to the other example, this mother-in-law was pushing her opinion onto her daughter-in-law with a harsh tone. But, María shrugged it off and replied that she was indeed complying with expected and appropriate dietary practices.

Mothers-in-law also played a role in decision-making for older women but in food benefits and cravings, and not for taboos. The finding that mothers-in-law continue to play a role in the construction of human agency and prenatal dietary practices is not surprising, as anthropological and sociological studies have focused on this relationship in the cross-cultural literature. Mothers-in-law are shown to be influential regarding various aspects of the pregnancy, such as prenatal care (White et al. 2013; Simkhada et al. 2010) and birth location (Ono et al. 2013; Sychareun et al. 2012).

There are a few scenarios involving mothers–in-law that are exemplary of Ortner's (1997) construct of serious games, which I argue can be framed as "serious games of reproduction." It has been well documented in the literature in physical anthropology that different individuals often have a stake in the rearing of young (Hrdy 2009). This could be due to a genetic link, in which the individual wants to propagate its own genetic line, or could be for other reasons, as Sarah Hrdy (2009) outlines in her book on cooperative breeding. Whatever the reason, the discipline could benefit from using Ortner's serious games model to explore the social relationships involved in reproduction and how these relationships shape human agency and decision-making during the perinatal period.

During two of my interviews mothers-in-law were present and it became clear that they provided a lot of material support for pregnant women to make sure that they were eating properly. This makes sense from a biological perspective, as relatives would want to ensure the survival of their offspring. Although one participant was clearly annoyed by the comments of her mother-in-law during the interview, she reluctantly agreed with her. I wondered why she would engage in this behavior, as she already had a child of her own, indicating that she had experiential knowledge. She also had a job and lived apart from her in-laws with her partner on the other side of town, indicating a degree of independence. As Ortner (1997) explains, actors participating in serious games "play with skill, intention, wit, knowledge, intelligence" (Loc.191). I argue that that she was most likely putting up with her mother-in-law's comments because she acted as a support system, which provided food and childcare. This seemed to be reflected in another case where the mother-in-law continually cut off her daughter-in-law during the interview to provide her own opinions. This mother-in-law was housing her daughter-in-law and providing her with food and other resources. These examples are conjecture since I was unable to gather the firsthand data needed to conduct a thorough analysis using this framework. However, they can still be used as examples and warrant further investigation using Ortner's framework to better understand maternal decision-making in contexts of rapidly shifting nutritional environments.

For women with older children, nineteen social actors were discussed within their narratives. In addition to most of the social actors mentioned earlier (except kids), father-in-law, employer, midwives, and older women were also mentioned by women with older children. The social actors mentioned by the most women with older children were mothers, partners, the clinic doctor, friends, and grandparents. In contrast to pregnant women, women with older children talked about many more social actors as they discussed all decision-making related constructs, including the doctor, grandparents, mothers, and mothers-in-law who seemed to play a role in various aspects of human agency (see tables 7.2 and 7.3).

Older women learned about prenatal dietary practices from their mothers and grandmothers, such as taboos against drinking chamomile tea, young coconut milk, and against eating spicy foods. One older woman noted, "That's what my mother told me, not to eat spicy peppers a lot because when the baby is born, the baby will be born and come out really burned" (Lucía, 45). Older women also got advice about food benefits, such as drinking milk for the calcium and to make their bones and the bones of their baby strong. Women with older children's diets were also constrained by what their mothers or the family could provide. Lucía went on to say, "In that time, more than anything it was the family. In the family if there was something that they had, what do I know, something from the harvest, my mom had milk so she would make sour cream. Things like that basically we would share." Advice also came from other women, such as grandmothers and aunts. One woman with older children said,

> Yes, my mother, and yes, the grandmothers, and the aunts. They always said, "if you are pregnant you should drink orange juice with an egg yolk every day. Since you have a lot of oranges, make a little orange juice." A friend and I made orange juice and she put the whole egg in. But she wasn't pregnant. And I said, "uyyy, how gross!" She told me, "no, you don't know anything, drink it!" So I looked for a small egg and I threw away the white and brought another glass and made a little bit of orange juice and I added the egg yolk and with the other glass with more juice in my hand and I went outside and I felt like I was going to burst. And afterwards I drank the rest of the juice. That is what we did almost everyday. (Samantha, 60)

In some cases this advice led to resistance against cultural norms. Although most women indicated that flaxseed could cause miscarriages, one woman with older children noted, "Yes. I drank a lot of flaxseed. People told me, 'be careful because they say that flaxseed is abortive.' And my grandmother always told us, 'no.' My grandmother had 14 children. Yes, I believe that there were 13 or 14 kids. Yes, 14 kids. Three deaths. But my grandmother always drank all that. And, yes, she told us, that plant, it doesn't seem to be true, that it is poisonous" (Abigail, 41). Three women's grandmothers were midwives and they respected the advice they received from them. "Only

Table 7.2 Social Actors and Human Agency among Women with Older Children I

	Partner (n=18)		*Clinic Doctor (n=6)*		*Grandparents (n=3)*	
	Instance of Overlap in Narrative	*C-coefficient*	*Instance of Overlap in Narrative*	*C-coefficient*	*Instance of Overlap in Narrative*	*C-coefficient*
Intentionality	7	.05	7	.05	7	.05
Negotiation	10	.07	6	.05	8	.07
Reproduction	X	X	7	.05	11	.08
Resistance	X	X	4	.07	6	.11

Table 7.3 Social Actors and Human Agency among Women with Older Children II

	Mother-in-Law (n=20)		*Mother (n=18)*	
	Instance of Overlap in Narrative	*C-coefficient*	*Instance of Overlap in Narrative*	*C-coefficient*
Intentionality	7	.06	14	.08
Negotiation	X	X	18	.11
Reproduction	X	X	X	X
Resistance	X	X	6	.06

through experience. She did it [midwifery] only through experience. It was incredible, my grandmother was incredible. She was like a doctor without studying. And she was very knowledgeable" (Alma, 41). Although the role of the clinic was already discussed above, some women with older children indicated doctors always knew best. "The doctors told you what best nutrition is" (Melissa, 51).

Chapter 8

Tourism and Culture Change

The evidence presented in this book shows a clear link between increased tourism and related development in the Monteverde Zone and features of the nutrition transition. Free listing participants specifically associated economic factors as influencing nutrition, and interview respondents mentioned that the tourism economy and dietary delocalization (often considered a catalyst of the nutrition transition) played a role as well. Survey respondents (n=52) believed that tourism influences what people eat in the Monteverde Zone through two mechanisms: "cultural influences" and "work."

CULTURAL INFLUENCES

Cultural influences included bringing more variety of foods and healthier habits to the region, such as increased knowledge about healthier foods (e.g., Quinoa and salads) and increased access to fast foods and junk foods (e.g., pizza and hamburgers), which are incorporated into the local setting as part of the "tourist diet." These are the same foods that participants indicated are junk foods and are categorized as unhealthy, or contributing to poor nutrition. One participant noted, "Ticos, many take on customs from others very easily: it doesn't have to be bad but sometimes it's not that healthy. Ticos have maintained a healthy diet for many years. Yes, the diet could be changed, but it shouldn't change because of fast food because it's not healthy" (male, 38 years old). Tourism research shows that the relationship between tourism and culture takes many forms (e.g., culture as a commodity), although it is clear that there is always an impact on local culture as a result of tourism (Bleasdale 2006). As Bleasdale (2006) notes, tourism can lead to acculturation for the host community. This is referred to as the "demonstration effect," in which locals imitate tourists in regards to clothing, language, lifestyle, or food choices (Fisher 2004). Acculturation is a common topic for studies exploring globalization and dietary quality (Himmelgreen et al. 2014) and studies on migration and diet have found that as migrants adopt a more "Western" diet, with characteristics similar to the nutrition transition, the changes can have both positive and negative impacts on dietary quality (Kleiser et al. 2010; Hammar et al. 2009). This fits with the fifth stage of the nutrition transition, where conscious behavioral change takes place to improve nutrition (Dufour and Bender 2013). Other research has shown that culinary traditions may be strengthened by tourism, as it is common for tourists to seek out authentic cultural traditions, including food customs (Mak et al. 2012; Bleasdale 2006; Wilk 1999). This was also reflected by one interview participant, who noted that local food traditions are still dominant in the Monteverde Zone because tourists want an authentic experience. Another participant noted that food culture among rural populations is consistent and stable and that is why many people in the Monteverde Zone still consume a traditional diet.

WORK

Although most survey participants recognized that tourism brings work to the Monteverde Zone, this was viewed as both positive and negative. It was positive because with work households could afford to purchase more food and healthier foods. However, participants recognized that with more work individuals have less time and may eat more junk foods or fast foods because it is easier and quicker. In contrast, interview participants indicated that the tourism economy is associated with work, diet, food prices, and food access. While only nine pregnant women in the sample were working at the time of the interview, seven of those women self-identified with working in tourism. Three of the women worked in supermarkets, three worked in a restaurant, one worked in a hotel, one worked in a store that she and her husband owned, and one worked as an operator for a local taxi company, working on average forty-three hours per week. All of the pregnant women indicated that someone else in the household was working at the time of data collection. The majority of which, worked in tourism. Five participants had two individuals in the home who were working, and of those, four worked in tourism. An important point to note is that for some participants who indicated that they didn't work, or that they didn't work in tourism, they still hosted multiple homestay students throughout the year, with a timeframe from a few days to a few months. Additionally, through participant observation some women sold makeup products or Amway products in the community. When asked if they worked, they said that they didn't but I later found out that they sold these products for money. Although this is beyond the scope of this work, it is important to recognize that locally constructed definitions of what constitutes work is important to take into consideration when exploring the impacts of shifting political economy on community well-being.

Across the sample, tourism was associated with employment. This included construction work from building tourism-related infrastructure (e.g., hotels, restaurants, stores, etc.) and direct work in the service industry (e.g., hotels, tours, etc.). As one pregnant woman noted, "So, it affects the economy already because it is a place that depends on tourism, if there is not tourism, there is no work. So employment goes down, salaries go down, everything goes down" (María, 18, 6 months pregnant). This also changed with the tourism season. Another pregnant woman said, "And, well, not everyone has work during that time, in the low season. Let's see, here is an example: my sister works in a hotel. During the low season she doesn't work. And, similarly, she has kids and her husband, but it's not the same as in high season. Her husband, let's say, in low season, yes, he works, but let's say it's half time. There are days when he has work and days when he doesn't" (Sofía, 22, 7.5 months pregnant). There was also consensus that as families and individuals began to rely more heavily on the tourism industry for work, they began to purchase more food, leaving agricultural production in favor of store-bought food items. As one woman with older children explained, "I think that having money sometimes makes it easier for people to go to the supermarket than to grind corn themselves, right" (Samantha, 60).

In the Monteverde Zone, the tourism economy has grown drastically since the early 1990s (Honey 2008), and now the mixed local economy is heavily dependent on tourism. Some 32 percent (n=7) of pregnant women were working in the tourism industry at the time of the interview. This is higher than national average, which estimate that 19.9 percent of Costa Ricans work in tourism (direct and indirectly) (ICT 2018). Although pregnant women worked forty-three hours a week, well within the legal Costa Rican limits (forty-eight hours a week) (Asamblea Legislativa 1943), some pregnant women worked upward of seventy-seven hours during the busy season. The schedules affected dietary practices, as some pregnant women expressed difficulty in finding time to eat regularly during working hours, and some noted that it was challenging to take care of themselves outside of work as they were exhausted from working long hours. As older women noted, dietary practices in the region have changed as people today tend to go for quicker and more easily prepared processed foods, including prepared drink mixes and packaged meats. This is similar to another study from the area, which found that 5.8 percent of the sample (n=200) noted the effect of shifting work patterns on dietary choices (Himmelgreen et al. 2014). Women found that their schedules conflicted with local store hours, making it hard to purchase

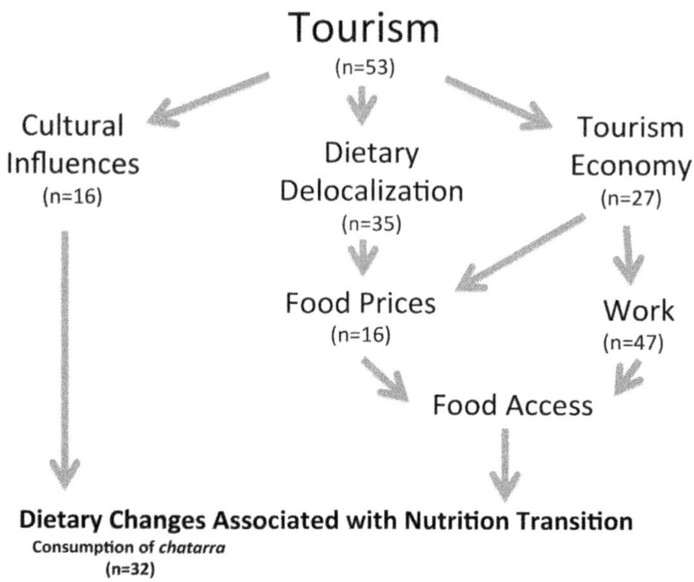

Figure 8.1 Tourism and Culture Change.

foods and that they were turning to fast foods and easily prepared foods (e.g., hamburgers and hot dogs) as they didn't have as much time as they used to. Links between women working in tourism and negative impacts on dietary behaviors have been noted elsewhere in the literature (Nakamura et al. 2002), as work in tourism often involves long work hours to fit the demands of the tourists schedules (Bauer 2008), and women are often still required to maintain domestic duties in addition to their work outside of the home (Gentry 2007; Cukier et al. 1996). Interview participants indicated that tourism influences dietary changes associated with the nutrition transition through work, food prices, and food access (see figure 8.1).

FOOD ACCESS AND FOOD PRICES

Increased dietary delocalization (Pelto and Pelto 1983) in the Monteverde Zone was associated with food prices and food access through the development of infrastructure. This occurred through improvements made to the main road that connects the community with the Pan-American Highway, as well as the opening of two chain supermarkets. The paving of the road is currently underway. The improvements made so far have made it easier to bring food into the community. This includes fresh foods (e.g., fruits and vegetables) and packaged and processed foods that are part of the larger industrial food system. Two important examples stand out in regards to this. First, as the previously community-owned cheese factory is now part of the Mexican company, Sigma (Sigma 2019), large trucks travel up the mountain day and night to bring products such as Yoplait yogurt and Del Prado cheese, as well as Monteverde Cheese Factory products that are now produced elsewhere. Additionally, the local supermarkets sell poultry from Pipasa, a large Costa Rican company, which was bought by the U.S.-based global conglomerate corporation Cargill in 2011 (Cargill Incorporated 2015). Cargill has been operating in Costa Rica since 1999, when it purchased Cinta Azul, a Costa Rican company that makes packaged sandwich meats. Participants agreed that as more community members opted to participate in the tourism economy there was less food production in the region as a whole, and an overall increase in the reliance on store-bought food items. This pattern was documented by other researchers in the area (Himmelgreen et al. 2014, 2006) and has been noted in other regions of Latin America (Reardon et al. 2005; Dewey 1989; Caballero 1984). One prominent example is from Mexico, where there are accounts that in tourism regions some households have abandoned local food production in favor of increased participation in the market economy, which limits the amount of time individuals and families have to produce, process, and prepare foods (Leatherman et al. 2010; Leatherman and Goodman 2005). The increased reliance on store-bought foods can be problematic when there are issues with food quality. As Ruiz (2014) points out, differential growth patterns between children in food secure and food insecure households in the Monteverde Zone may be due to difference in dietary quality, as the children in food secure households showed higher rates of stunting. Although the households were food secure, diet quality may account for this inverse and paradoxical relationship.

It has been well documented that the addition of grocery stores in communities which previously did not have them changes local dietary practices, as this increases access to a wider variety of foods (Asfaw 2008; Moore et al. 2008; Morland et al. 2006). Although the Monteverde Zone had one supermarket prior to the rapid tourism-driven development, the addition of major chain stores has increased the variety of foods that are available. In Guatemala, Asfaw (2008) found that after supermarkets appeared participants began to include processed and packaged foods in the diet as a replacement for some staple items. This fits with the data presented here, as street-intercept survey participants indicated that new work patterns limited the time they had for food preparation, and therefore they consumed increased amounts of junk foods and fast foods due to their affordability and easy and quick preparation. These types of foods are available through fast food restaurants and supermarkets in the Monteverde Zone. Others have noted the positive increase in dietary quality with the appearance of supermarkets, especially in the United

States (Moore et al. 2008; Morland et al. 2006). Survey participants also indicated that increased employment opportunities that came with growing infrastructure (e.g., construction work and jobs in tourism) allowed individuals to purchase healthier foods and larger quantities of foods. However, as Drewnowski and colleagues (2012) indicate, it may not be the presence of grocery stores alone that influences dietary practices, but cost may also play a role. As mentioned throughout the sample, the economy was a factor that participants felt contributed to getting adequate nutrition, as food prices in the region were considered to be high and work was often seasonal. This seasonality affects dietary decision-making because, as Himmelgreen and colleagues (2006) pointed out, in the Monteverde Zone "the tourist season goes down, but not the prices." Participants linked the high prices of food with the fact that foods come from outside the region, and pregnant women noted that some foods are more expensive when the tourism season is low (e.g., meat) and people typically have less to spend.

TOURISM AND FOOD ACCESS

Another common theme emerged that indicated tourism influenced food access through seasonality of tourism and the relationship between tourism and food prices. There is a negotiation with the growing season and the tourism season, which can result in less access to certain foods if production is lower due to work in the tourism industry. As one older woman noted,

> When there are a lot of tourists the hotels buy all the fruit. Because of this, it's easier to access foods in the low tourism season. There is also a difference in the price of food. For example, meat is more expensive when the tourist season is low since local meat producers change their prices based on the prices found in the supermarkets.

According to participants, the supermarkets raise their prices for meat in the low season, which sets the selling price for local producers as well. This makes it harder to purchase some items when the tourist season is low.
Participants mentioned the difficulty in purchasing both meat and fruit during the low season. Additionally, there are more sales during high tourist season, which means lower prices. As one pregnant woman said,

> Yes, yes it affects it. For example, when there is a high level of tourism, in general it's easier. Okay, at first for us when there is a lot of tourism, we have the option of giving a homestay to students, so it's extra money that comes into the house. So, it's better. In general, when there is a lot of tourism, then there are more sales, then there is more competition in between the businesses and

> they have to lower their prices because people might prefer that other place. But, when the season is low, there aren't people, so we can't give anyone a homestay. And that money is not coming in. So the markets, in case they can't sell, they will have more sales so that they can get rid of products and others that raise the prices because there is not a lot of product and because they know that people need that product, and because there isn't a lot they are going to buy it at whatever price. So, yes, yes it affects us a lot when there is tourism and when there isn't very much tourism. (Maricella, 25, 3 months pregnant)

There were a couple of respondents (n=2) who said that there was no influence of the seasonality of tourism or that it only affects you if you work in tourism, since less work equals less money to purchase food.

PRENATAL FOOD SECURITY

Food access is one dimension of food insecurity that has already been researched in this community. In light of previous National Science Foundation–funded research in the area that reported high rates of food insecurity, I also measured food insecurity among pregnant women's households. Although most pregnant women I spoke with were food secure (n=13), some were mildly food insecure (n=4) and others were moderately food insecure (n=3). None experienced severe household food insecurity. I used the household food insecurity access scale (HFIAS)[1] to assess food insecurity in this setting, which has been used to measure household food insecurity during the perinatal period in various settings (Jebena et al. 2015; Bartelink et al. 2014; Young et al. 2014; Dewing et al. 2013; Gebremedhin et al. 2011).

The rates of food insecurity described here are much lower than those found by past researchers in the region. Himmelgreen and colleagues (2006) found that among 148 households, food insecurity was between 67 percent and 73 percent, whereas only 35 percent of households were food insecure in this study. Additional research conducted by Himmelgreen and colleagues (2014) found that among 215 households, 50.7 percent were food insecure. As these studies were conducted over the span of fifteen years, it is possible that food insecurity within this community is decreasing, as residents adapt to their shifting food environments and the change in political economy, which has occurred with the transition to a tourism-driven job market. It is also possible that due to this study's much smaller sample size that there is less variation in food security status overall, or there was some characteristic of pregnant women who chose to participate in the study that made them more food secure. A third possibility, is that the presence of a pregnant woman in the household may be a factor in household food security status, as everyone recognizes that prenatal nutrition is important and that women should be taken care of during this time. This is evidenced by the interactions between women and their mothers-in-law (which has been discussed in the preceding chapters), who continually purchase foods and prepare foods for the well-being of their daughters-in-law and unborn grandchildren. Additionally, one participant noted that an older woman at her work would bring her snacks and check in on her frequently. The food insecurity literature indicates that there is sometimes a buffering effect for children (Piperata et al. 2013; Melgar-Quinonez et al. 2008; Oldewage-Theron et al. 2006) and people with disabilities (Corman et al. 2014), although to the best of my knowledge there is no work being done to explore this trend among pregnant women.

Women themselves had a lot of knowledge about what types of food they should be eating and would cope with high food prices and lower availability of food items, to curb food insecurity, in various ways, such as purchasing foods (e.g., kiwis) outside of the Monteverde Zone where they were cheaper and there was more variety. It is unclear if they would go to such lengths even if they were not pregnant, as many in the community have discussed the need to leave the Monteverde Zone to purchase cheaper foods (Himmelgreen et al. 2014).

Some of the trends identified in the statistical analysis (not presented in this book)[2] fit with the literature on food insecurity, such as the trend between body mass index and food insecurity, and number of hours worked and food insecurity, which have been noted elsewhere (Franklin et al. 2012; Coleman-Jensen 2011). Interestingly, saturated fat intake was high among most pregnant women in the sample and there was a statistically significant relationship between saturated fat intake and food security. The greatest contributors to saturated fat intake were meat (32%), sweets (18%), and cheese (13%). Although these items are readily available in the area, they may not be considered "staple" items, as rice and beans might be, leading the more food secure households to have a better chance at accessing them when they have the resources to do so. Additionally, as participants mentioned the high prices of meat (especially in the low season), it is possible that more food secure households have greater access to meats because of financial resources. Another possibility is that households are sacrificing dietary quality and opting to purchase cheaper, more processed meats. This second possibility would fit with findings by Ruiz (2014), which were described previously.

Tourism, Diet, and Nutrition

There was also the recognition that tourism is linked with dietary behaviors. As individuals integrate further into the tourist/market economy, they have the ability to purchase more food items, which changes the traditional diet in many ways. As one pregnant woman noted,

> The zone in which we live is an area that has too much influence from tourism. It has been acculturated a lot, so already there are families that don't worry too much about conserving, let's say, the indigenous recipes for everything, so the famous "fast foods" or many recipes that have been included in the daily diet, let's say, from the families. It's easier to get a box of hamburger patties from the refrigerator than to buy the meat and make the patty, for example. (Melina, 33, 7 months pregnant)

Additionally, the increased accessibility of food from outside the region increases dietary delocalization. With more people working in tourism there is less agricultural production and increased reliance on store-bought food items. One older woman, Melissa (51), indicated that if you grow food then you always have something, but as many aren't growing anymore, access to food is changing. There is also a link with fast food restaurants that have opened and purchasing of different, more processed food items, such as processed meats. Beyond working in the service industry, many women in the sample talked about the influence of the homestay students on their own diet and that of their families. However, interview participants did note that customs and daily eating habits are changing, especially with the influence of tourism. As one pregnant woman discussed the influence of having students in their home, she said, "And, yes, it helps us a lot because we have changes a lot of our dietary habits since we have had students, so there are things that we didn't eat before and because we had the foods for the students we began to eat them and we liked them, so it's a custom or habit that has stayed in the house or for the family to eat" (Maricella, 25, 3 months pregnant). Maricella went on to say,

> And after we had students we ate more vegetables. We try to eat less rice. Before we would maybe prepare rice, beans and pasta. Now if I make pasta, we only eat pasta, so it's not so much carbohydrates. . . . If there is fish, we will make a salad and fish, or chicken and salad, or chicken and vegetables. Then we don't eat rice. So, yes it has helped us a lot, and the kids have learned to eat more things that they didn't want before, but to see that in the family it's a habit or custom to eat it, for them it's what is made.

Similarly, some others indicated that tourism brought positive dietary changes to the region. Some participants noted that there is actually better nutrition in Monteverde Zone because of tourism, since compared with other places in Costa Rica people in the Monteverde Zone eat healthier because of the tourist influence, this also has to do with higher socioeconomic status than other places. One older woman said,

> Maybe, yes, because, for example in Monteverde, with it being a tourist area, I think that there is better nutrition than in other places in the country that don't have tourism, because for example there are people that visit us from maybe San Jose or Alajuela and they say, but, what is this? I'm not familiar with this. What is this food?' It's like you, maybe, how would I say it, it's like eating food that is more natural. We have, let's say . . . here in Monteverde the people look for food that is the most natural as possible, that doesn't have a lot of chemicals, that is hopefully grown in the zone. In contrast, you go to other places and everything is purchased from the supermarket. Maybe everything is prepared in a restaurant or frozen. In Monteverde the tourism has made the people grow more, to have more traditional foods for tourists, so the people, let's say, are used to these foods. (Clara, 33)

One example is access to healthier foods that tourists want, such as granola. One participant noted that her family in Tilarán (a community about an hour and a half away) had never heard of granola, but that she started eating it because of the tourist influence.

Overall, participants agreed that there is also a cultural influence occurring and that the desire for specific foods changes as locals want to eat the foods that tourists want to eat. "I think that, I don't know, it's like a way to copy another person, or thinking that this is more interesting, things that come from outside, externally. Or that the food of Costa Rica is more boring, like many people say. So, we are trying to copy others" (Melina, 33, 7 months pregnant). When probed about if this influence was coming from the foreigners that come here or from the media she responded, "I think a little bit of everything always influences the cultural part and this shapes how we live today."

TOURISM AND THE NUTRITION TRANSITION

It is clear from the research presented in this book that a nutrition transition has occurred in the Monteverde Zone. However, impacts on pregnancy diet appeared to be minimal. It is possible that large-scale changes brought on by tourism and the nutrition transition have already occurred and become part of the "typical" diet, making it hard to identify a stark contrast in dietary practices over the previous generation. Evidence from the interviews with older women show that in the past it was more difficult to purchase items, as there was no formal road in and out of the community, and the main form of transportation was horseback. These women also indicated that most of what they ate came from the food they grew or animals they raised. However, they did report purchasing staple items such as rice and oil even when they had to leave the Monteverde Zone in order to do so. Based on this evidence, it's possible that the incorporation of higher fat items (with the purchase cooking oils) and added sugars and refined carbohydrates (with the purchase of store-bought goods) occurred many years ago, and that some of these foods may have already been adopted as part of regional and typical dietary practices. Additionally, the arrival of the Quakers in 1951 probably had an impact on local dietary behaviors, although there is currently no data from the region to explore this claim. It is also possible that the actual regional dishes haven't changed since tourism has increased, but that access to foods has. As there was a link between tourism and work as described by participants, there may be increased access to cash, which would allow participants to purchase some items (e.g., meats) more frequently than in the past. As mentioned previously, the presence of supermarkets has the potential to improve dietary quality. Laraia and colleagues (2004) explored this hypothesis among pregnant women and found that living closer to a supermarket improved dietary quality within their sample. Another interpretation of the findings presented in this study is that the reliance on store-bought food items has helped to ensure a higher diet quality among pregnant women. Abu-Saad and colleagues (2012) also noted the decreased reliance on traditional homemade items by pregnant women in the context of the nutrition transition. However, in contrast to the results presented here, Abu-Saad and colleagues (2012) found a high rate of dietary deficiencies (e.g., protein intake and dietary fiber) associated with this finding. Although this research was conducted in a very different setting (among a Bedouin population that has recently become more sedentary), its contribution to exploring the relationship between the nutrition transition and prenatal nutrition is worth noting.

TOURISM AND HUMAN AGENCY

Within the sample there was no relationship between tourism and any constructs of human agency or dietary practices This is surprising, as the other data indicate that tourism is intimately involved with food access and shifting food environments in the Monteverde Zone (through the economy, work, and cultural forces). It is possible that tourism has an indirect relationship with dietary practices, as other data show the ways that tourism has influenced the food environment in the Monteverde Zone. I argue that this relationship is being mediated by deeply embedded cultural forces, as well as local dietary customs, and the desire to continue to engage in "the usual" dietary behaviors.

NOTES

1. HFIAS data were used to calculate two food security measurements, an overall food security scale score and a food insecurity access prevalence, which places each household in a food security category. The HFIAS scale score produces a score of food insecurity on a scale of 0 to 27. This number is produced by summing the

frequency of occurrence responses that correspond to each of the nine questions. Additionally, an indicator was calculated by using the mean scale score for the entire sample. The food insecurity access prevalence was also calculated, which grouped households into one of four levels: food secure, mild food insecurity, moderate food insecurity, or severe food insecurity. Levels are assigned based on a basic algorithm described by Coates and colleagues (2007).

2. In order to explore the relationship between food insecurity and categorical variables, a chi-square analysis (Field 2009) was conducted using food security status categories (i.e., food secure or food insecure). To explore the relationship between food security and nutritional status, a Spearman's rho (Field 2009) was conducted using the raw HFIAS food security score. Additionally, a Mann-Whitney U test (Field 2009) was conducted to explore differences in interval data by food security status (i.e., food secure or food insecure). Nonparametric tests were chosen because many of the variables were not normally distributed. Before running analysis all interval-level variables were tested for normality, first by visually inspecting the data on a histogram and then by examining levels of skewness and kurtosis. If variables exhibited either skewness (<-1/2 or > 1/2) or kurtosis (<-1/2 or > 1/2) (Field 2009) they were not normally distributed. Test results with a p value $\leq .05$ were considered statistically significant.

Conclusion

Why Practice Matters

A long-standing general critique of the research process is the exclusion of local voices, wherein the people under study lack the ability to speak for themselves (Wang 1999). This ultimately muffles the results, as researchers filter these voices through analysis and synthesis of the subject realities in the context of their research questions. This book presents the lived experiences of rural residents in the Monteverde Zone as they grapple with shifts in the food environment spurred on by tourism-impelled development since the 1990s.

Despite living in an increasingly globalized community, residents of the Monteverde Zone had a shared understanding of nutrition. This culturally constructed domain reflects a web of historical, social, and contemporary forces that work in concert to reinforce what it means to be Costa Rican. The importance placed on rice and beans within the sample illustrates this. At the same time the results show a high level of awareness about how nutrition can impact health, showing how this region may be set apart from others in the country because of high levels of education and the constant presence of international residents. Free listing data (n=52), semi-structured interviews (n=42), and focus groups (N=2, n=15) indicate that nutrition is a cultural construct which is part of shared national and regional identity.

This ultimately shaped ideas about prenatal diet and buffered pregnant women from the negative impacts of the nutrition transition. The results from the twenty-four-hour diet recalls show that pregnant women did not consume many foods characteristic of the nutrition transition and experienced low levels of food insecurity. Instead, they chose to maintain a diet that was *lo normal*, or the usual for the region, including the daily consumption of rice and beans. Shared beliefs also contributed to the ways that pregnant women viewed food taboos, prescriptions, and cravings during pregnancy.

For example, even though the belief that consuming soda would lead to a splotchy-skinned baby is not rooted in scientific evidence, women avoided sodas nonetheless, conferring some degree of protection from diets typical of the nutrition transition. Other beliefs, such as the notion that consuming chamomile tea will lead to miscarriage are seemingly false, but are rooted in local knowledge that does hold up under scientific scrutiny and should be respected.

Shared ideas about nutrition in general and prenatal dietary practices played a role in women's decision-making (n=42), although this was juxtaposed with changes over time, which included differences in food access and social actors. While increased access to various food sources was noted as an important feature of contemporary life in the Monteverde Zone, the high food prices played a role in decision-making on where to shop and what to buy. Pregnant women identified fewer social actors who were influential when it came to dietary decision-making (16 vs. 24 for older women). However, the mother-in-law consistently played a role in prenatal decision-making regarding food choices. This reflects the steadfast nature of some aspect of local culture despite widespread changes to the social fabric of everyday life in the region after the tourism boom.

I argue that nuanced research (such as the work presented here) is imperative to assessing maternal health in a global society, where rapid environmental changes are juxtaposed with traditional practices. Overall, this work makes major contributions to theory building efforts at the intersection of anthropology and public health. I have used practice theory in a way which strengthens the relationship between theory and methods and has practical implications for the field of maternal health.

THEORY

Practice Theory

Throughout this book I argue for the importance of using practice theory and examine actual practices in order to understand the impacts of the global nutrition transition on prenatal health in the Monteverde Zone, Costa Rica. From the evidence presented, it is clear that the shift in local foodways has not impacted pregnancy health in any apparent way, although the processes underlying constructs of human agency (i.e., intentionality, reproduction, resistance, negotiation) (Ortner 1997) relevant to decision-making have shifted over time. This is an important finding, as it sheds light on the nuanced ways that change occurs. Even more pertinent to the discussion here is the methodology I use to identify these aspects of change. I operationalize practice theory in a way that is feasible and reproducible. This makes a novel contribution to the way that data is collected and addresses one of the major challenges in conducting community-level qualitative research: time. While this type of research enables investigators to explore local, lived realities, it also takes a considerable about of time to build rapport and earn trust within communities. I argue that developing streamlined and validated methods that integrate theory and practice will help researchers working at the community level to produce high-quality comparable data that can better inform community and national maternal health policies. These policies are often guided by trends in global data that do not take into account the distinctions for regional and subregional populations. In chapter 4 (Expanding the Nutrition Transition), I describe my methodology for applying practice theory (more details are provided in the endnotes) in the hopes that others will do the same. Having a broad base of this type of comparable data will reveal more about how humans react to change than large-scale quantitative analysis can because, as anthropologists have pointed out for decades, variation is a key feature of humanity. One way I would improve this methodology for future use would be to gather baseline data on constructs of human agency at the community level to develop consensus within a local context in regards to what exactly constitutes "negotiation," "intentionality," "reproduction," and "resistance."

The Nutrition Transition

This book contributes to the nutrition transition literature in two significant ways. First, as the research on the direct links between tourism and the nutrition transition are limited, this book has helped to fill some of that paucity. Understanding the relationship between tourism development and dietary change is important since the world is more connected than ever before, which makes tourism more accessible. Tourism development results in rapid changes that affect local communities, as well as the tourists that visit them. Second, there is a dearth in the literature regarding the association between the nutrition transition and prenatal dietary practices. In this case study, cultural factors played a strong role in mediating this relationship, resulting in a minimal effect during the prenatal period. This finding contradicts other literature, which did find impacts on prenatal diet as a result of the nutrition transition (Abu-Saad et al. 2012), highlighting the need for more work in this area. While the women in this book consumed adequate prenatal diets in the context of the nutrition transition, others report similar findings for subpopulations and attribute this to the early stages of the nutrition transition (Dalzell et al. 2017). Further, the finding that there may be various stages of the nutrition transition occurring at the same time (i.e., nutrition-related chronic noncommunicable diseases and positive behavioral changes) in this region indicates that applying a population-level framework to local settings could be problematic, especially when it comes to health prevention and intervention strategies.

The Critical Biocultural Approach

This study also contributes to the literature on the CBCA in anthropology, as the application of practice theory in this book was in response to the recognition that human agency was often missing from studies on the nutrition transition (Popkin et al. 2012) and research that employs the CBCA (Leatherman and Goodman 2011). As discussed earlier, practice theory makes a much-needed contribution to biocultural studies by providing a framework through which to apply an agency-oriented approach and through the use of firsthand observations of behavior (versus reported behavior). Although there were limitations on applying practice theory in this study,[1] the findings on the interaction between human agency and other environmental influences (e.g., social actors) highlight the complexities inherent to the ways the communities and subpopulations cope with environmental changes. In this case, the strong cultural identity of being pregnant in this region buffered women from the negative health consequences of the nutrition transition. However, an analysis of the ways that human agency is constructed within this context shows the various pathways that women take to make decisions related to prenatal diet. To the best of my knowledge, this is the first study to analyze constructs of human agency in relationship to decision-making over time in the context of shifting nutritional environments. Applying this additional level of analysis to understanding biological data (e.g., nutritional status) provides an in-depth analytical framework for understanding how environmental changes impact (or fail to impact) specific populations. While most studies employing the CBCA rely on a description of the phenomena taking place, this case study identifies the underlying processes that guide decision-making, providing a foundation for understanding prenatal health in the context of the nutrition transition in this setting. A recent edited volume describing contemporary studies in biocultural anthropology (Zuckerman and Martin 2016) also works to fill some of the historical gaps in applying the CBCA.

PRACTICAL IMPLICATIONS FOR MATERNAL HEALTH

In Costa Rica, maternal health indicators are closer to those of more developed and industrialized nations than in the neighboring region. For example, Costa Rica's maternal mortality ratio is 21.2, while in comparison, the bordering countries of Nicaragua and Panama have ratios of 35.1 and 49.2 respectively (PAHO 2019). Despite being a global leader in healthcare, 59.9 percent of

Costa Ricans are overweight (24% are obese) (WHO 2016). For women, this number is 61.9 percent (WHO 2016). This book shows the important role that culture plays in guiding dietary behaviors. It's unclear what diet and health behaviors were for the women before their pregnancies (or after), but it is apparent that a sense of cultural identity shaped women's decision-making processes and dietary behaviors during pregnancy. This has important implications in light of the developmental origins of health and disease theory. During pregnancy, the fitness of both the mother and the developing fetus are dependent on the same pool of resources, indicating that trade-offs may occur between the two when resources are limited or compromised (e.g., inadequate or excessive intake of macronutrients and micronutrients). Fetal origins hypothesis, or commonly called the developmental origins of health and disease theory (DOHaD), explains that trade-offs occur in the fetus when the maternal environment is compromised in some way (e.g., inadequate nutrition). "The DOHaD concept describes how during early life (at conception, and/or during fetal life, infancy and early childhood), the environment induces changes in development that have long term impacts on later health and disease risk" (DOHaD Society 2013). DOHaD has established the link between nutritional perturbations during critical developmental windows and the propensity for disease risk in offspring, which can be inherited across generations (Bogin and Smith 2012; Barker 2012; Benyshek 2007; Gluckman and Hanson 2006). DOHaD research often focuses on measures of maternal nutritional stress experienced during pregnancy and their association with disease risk across the life course, including metabolic syndrome, overweight/obesity, cardiovascular disease, cognitive disorders, osteoporosis, cancer, type 2 diabetes, and hypertension (Hanson and Gluckman 2015; Barker 2012; Littleton et al. 2010; Kuzawa and Quinn 2009; Gluckman and Hanson 2008; Benyshek 2007; Bogin et al. 2007; Benyshek et al. 2006, 2001; McDade 2005; Painter et al. 2005; Roseboom et al. 2001; Barker et al. 1989; Barker and Osmond 1986). In addition to shifting diets and lifestyles linked with the nutrition transition, DOHaD provides an explanatory model that accounts for biological factors that contribute to propensity toward chronic noncommunicable disease across generations. The coupling of these phenomena (the nutrition transition and processes underlying nutritional perturbations during the perinatal period) may have contributed to the excessive increase in chronic noncommunicable diseases that has occurred on a global scale.

RECOMMENDATIONS

Among pregnant women in this sample prenatal dietary practices have not changed much over time, food insecurity is lower than reported by other studies, and nutritional and health status is adequate. However, as various constructs related to decision-making have changed over time and some foods associated with the nutrition transition were consumed among pregnant women, it is possible that changes experienced by the population at large may affect pregnant women in the future. Based on study findings that the family and the clinic are still important sources of information about prenatal dietary practices, these outlets should be targeted for education that aims to maintain nutrition and health status and prevent detrimental shifts in consumption among this subpopulation. Additionally, the mother-in-law seemed to play a role in decision-making, and therefore, education efforts should involve these social actors as well.

As this book shows, pregnant women were not impacted to a large extent by tourism or the nutrition transition in this region. This highlights the need to better understand how the nutrition transition, a population-based model, plays out in local settings, as the effects are not linear and uniform cross-culturally. I plan to collaborate with others working in rural Latin America to identify the ways in which the large-scale changes in the nutritional environment associated with the nutrition transition affect prenatal health. Gathering cross-cultural data in this way will provide a foundation of knowledge to better understand how communities cope with changes in the food environment, and will help to identify the similarities and differences in the ways that rural populations are affected by these shifts. I also plan to identify and utilize large datasets in Latin America that can be used to explore the relationship between the nutrition transition and perinatal nutritional and health status at the population level. It is important to understand how large-scale frameworks affect health among subpopulations in various regions of the world, as this type of work paves the way for prevention and intervention efforts.

In conclusion, this study established links among tourism, the nutrition transition, and diet change in the Monteverde Zone, although the relationship with prenatal diet was not as discernable. There was a strong cultural component to prenatal dietary practices, which included dietary customs (i.e., *costumbres*), local beliefs (i.e., *creencias*), and the desire to consume the "usual" Costa Rican fare (i.e., "lo normal"), which did not appear to be impacted directly by tourism. The construction of human agency regarding prenatal dietary practices has shifted over time to include fewer social actors in decision-making, although sources of information have remained similar. Overall, this study highlights the need to investigate the ways that population-level explanatory frameworks, such as the nutrition transition, play out at a local level.

Based on the overall findings from this study, it appears that the relationship between the shifting food environment, the nutrition transition, and dietary intake was mediated by local customs, beliefs, and the idea that participants were consuming a typical Costa Rican diet. Prenatal dietary practices were situated within what free listing participants identified as a culturally constructed idea of nutrition and associated food items (e.g., consumption of rice and beans). Further, some of these practices were influenced heavily by the local belief system (e.g., hot/cold disease theory) and were guided by the idea that pregnant women were consuming "lo normal," or, "the usual." Amid the fast-paced and rapidly changing global environment, this book shows that culture can act as a constant and mediating force. While this doesn't mean that all aspects of culture are protective, I argue that streamlining in-depth and nuanced community-level research can show how cultural systems contribute to resiliency in uncertain times.

NOTE

1. My positionality as a researcher within a community that is saturated with educators, students, and researchers was a barrier to recruitment, as many saw me as just another "researcher." This ultimately limited sample size, which placed certain constraints on the analysis.

Bibliography

Abu-Saad, Kathleen, Danit R. Shahar, Drora Fraser, Hillel Vardi, Michael Friger, Arkardy Bolotin, and Laurence S. Freedman. 2012. "Adequacy of usual dietary intake and nutritional status among pregnant women in the context of nutrition transition: The DEPOSIT study." *British Journal of Nutrition* 108 (10):1874–1883.

Ackerman, Sara L. 2010. "Plastic paradise: Transforming bodies and selves in Costa Rica's cosmetic surgery tourism industry." *Medical Anthropology* 29 (4):403–423.

ACOG. 2018. *Frequently Asked Questions FAQ001 Pregnancy: Nutrition during Pregnancy*. The American College of Obstetricians and Gynecologists.

Adams, Elizabeth J., Laurence Grummer-Strawn, and Gilberto Chavez. 2003. "Food insecurity is associated with increased risk of obesity in California women." *The Journal of Nutrition* 133 (4):1070–1074.

Adams, Maurianne, Warren J. Blumenfield, Camelita (Rosie) Castañeda, Heather W. Hackman, Madeline L. Peters, and Ximena Zúñiga, eds. 2013. *Readings for Diversity and Social Justice: An Anthology on Racism, Sexism, Anti-Semitism, Heterosexism Classism, and Ableism.* Edited by Maurianne Adams et al. New York; London: Routledge, 2000.

Agency, Central Intelligence. 2019. "The World Factbook." accessed March 5, 2019. https://www.cia.gov/library/publications/the-world-factbook/geos/cs.html.

Agüero, María Luisa Ávila. 2009. *Encuesta Nacional de Nutrición, Costa Rica, 2008–2009*. Ministerio de Salud, Instituto Costarricense de Investigación y Enseñanza en Nutrición y Salud, Caja Costarricense de Seguro Social, Instituto Nacional de Estadística y Censos, Instituto Costarricense sobre Drogas, INCAP/OPS.

Ahearn, Laura M. 2001. "Language and agency." *Annual Review of Anthropology* 30 (1) 109–137.

Ahlqvist, M., and E. Wirfalt. 2000. "Beliefs concerning dietary practices during pregnancy and lactation—A qualitative study among Iranian women residing in Sweden." *Scandinavian Journal of Caring Sciences* 14 (2):105–111. doi: 10.1080/02839310050162334.

Ajantha, Awnish K. Singh, Bhavya Malhotra, Surapaneni Krishna Mohan, and Ashish Joshi. 2015. "Evaluation of dietary choices, preferences, knowledge and related practices among pregnant women living in an Indian setting." *Journal of Clinical and Diagnostic Research: JCDR* 9 (8):LC04–10. doi: 10.7860/jcdr/2015/14463.6317.

Alarcón, Ana M. and Nahuelcheo S. Yolanda. 2008. "Pregnancy, delivery, and post partum beliefs among Mapuche women: Private conversations." *Chungara-Revista de Antropologia Chilena* 40 (2):193–202.

Albala, Cecilia, Fernando Vio, Juliana Kain, and Ricardo Uauy. 2001. "Nutrition transition in Latin America: The case of Chile." *Nutrition Reviews* 59 (6):170–176.

Ali, H. I., A. H. Jarrar, M. El Sadig, and K. B. Yeatts. 2013. "Diet and carbohydrate food knowledge of multi-ethnic women: A comparative analysis of pregnant women with and without gestational diabetes mellitus." *Plos One* 8 (9):9. doi: 10.1371/journal.pone.0073486.

Alimentos, Sigma. 2013. "Información Corporativa." http://www.sigma-alimentos.com/#home.

Alimentos, Sigma. 2019. "Información Corporativa." https://www.sigma-alimentos.com/brands-brochure.

Amuna, Paul, and Francis B. Zotor. 2008. "Epidemiological and nutrition transition in developing countries: Impact on human health and development." *Proceedings of the Nutrition Society* 67 (01):82–90. doi: doi:10.1017/S0029665108006058.

Angrosino, Michael, and Judith Rosenberg. 2011. "Observations on observation: Continuities and challenges." In *The Sage handbook of qualitative research*, edited by Norma K. Denzin and Yvonna S. Lincoln. Los Angeles: SAGE.

APA. 2019. "Diet during pregnancy." American Pregnancy Association. https://americanpregnancy.org/pregnancy-health/diet-during-pregnancy/.

Araya, Marlene Roselló, and Sonia Guzmán Padilla. 2004. "Trends in mortality from ischemic heart disease and acute myocardial infarction in Costa Rica, 1970–2001." *Revista Panamericana de Salud Pública* 16 (5):295–301.

Arias, L. 2014. "Costa Rica faces bean shortage, prompting emergency call for imports." *Tico Times*, Agriculture.

Armelagos, George J. and Alan H. Goodman. 1998. "Race, racism, and anthropology." In *Building a New Biocultural Synthesis: Political-Economic Perspectives on Human Biology*, edited by Alan H. and Thomas L. Leatherman Goodman, 359–378. Ann Arbor: University of Michigan Press.

Arps, Shahna. 2011. "Socioeconomic status and body size among women in Honduran Miskito communities." *Annals of Human Biology* 38 (4):508–519.

Arzoaquoi, S. K., E. E. Essuman, F. Y. Gbagbo, E. Y. Tenkorang, and I. Soyiri, and A.K. Laar. 2015. "Motivations for food prohibitions during pregnancy and their enforcement mechanisms in a rural Ghanaian district." *Journal of Ethnobiology and Ethnomedicine* 11:9. doi: 10.1186/s13002-015-0044-0.

Asfaw, Abay. 2008. "Does supermarket purchase affect the dietary practices of households? Some empirical evidence from Guatemala." *Development Policy Review* 26 (2):227–243.

Astrup, Arne, Jørn Dyerberg, Matthew Selleck, and, and Steen Stender. 2008. "Nutrition transition and its relationship to the development of obesity and related chronic diseases." *Obesity Reviews* 9:48–52. doi: 10.1111/j.1467-789X.2007.00438.x.

Aylward, Bruce, Katie Allen, Jaime Echeverría, and Joseph Tosi. 1996. "Sustainable ecotourism in Costa Rica: The Monteverde cloud forest preserve." *Biodiversity & Conservation* 5 (3):315–343.

Baer, Hans A. 1982. "On the political economy of health." *Medical Anthropology Newsletter* 14 (1):1–17.

Baer, Hans A. 1990. "Biocultural approaches in medical anthropology: A critical medical anthropology commentary." *Medical Anthropology Quarterly* 4 (3):344–348.

Baker, Scott, Janelle Elliot, Desirae Nasrallah, and Kenna Noone-Kirkpatrick. 2006. "The perceptions of waste water as an issue of public health importance in the Monteverde Zone, Costa Rica." In *Community Health 2006*. Monteverde: University of South Florida and the Monteverde Institute.

Bank, World. 2013. "Poverty headcount ratio at national poverty line (% of population)." The World Bank Group, accessed December 10, 2013. http://data.worldbank.org/country/costa-rica.

Banks, Tarika, Joshua Baxter, Austin Cox, Linda Gordon, and Deborah Robinson. 2010. "'Lo que mata, engorda': An exploratory profile of elderly nutrition in the Monteverde Region." In *Community Health 2010*. Monteverde: University of South Florida and the Monteverde Institute.

Barker, D.J.P. 2012. "Developmental origins of chronic disease." *Public Health* 126 (3):185–189. doi: http://dx.doi.org/10.1016/j.puhe.2011.11.014.

Barker, D.J.P. and C. Osmond. 1986. "Infant mortality, childhood nutrition, and ischaemic heart disease in England and Wales." *Lancet* 1.

Barker, David J.P., C. Osmond, P.D. Winter, B. Margetts, and S.J. Simmonds. 1989. "Weight in infancy and death from ischaemic heart disease." *The Lancet* 334 (8663):577–580.

Barrett, Ronald, Christopher W. Kuzawa, Thomas McDade, and George J. Armelagos. 1998. "Emerging and re-emerging infectious diseases: The third epidemiologic transition." *Annual Review of Anthropology* 27 (1) 247–271.

Bartelink, Imke H., Rada M. Savic, Julia Mwesigwa, Jane Achan, Tamara Clark, Albert Plenty, Edwin Charlebois, Moses Kamya, Sera L. Young, and Monica Gandhi. 2014. "Pharmacokinetics of Lopinavir/Ritonavir and Efavirenz in food insecure HIV-infected pregnant and breastfeeding women in Tororo, Uganda." *The Journal of Clinical Pharmacology* 54 (2):121–132.

Bauer, Irmgard. 2008. "The health impact of tourism on local and indigenous populations in resource-poor countries." *Travel Medicine and Infectious Disease* 6 (5):276–291.

Benyshek, D.C. 2007. "The development origins of obesity and related health disorders: Prenatal and perinatal sactors." *Collegium Anthropologicum* 31 (1):11–17.

Benyshek, D. C., C. S. Johnston, and J. F. Martin. 2006. "Glucose metabolism is altered in the adequately-nourished grand-offspring (F3 generation) of rats malnourished during gestation and perinatal life." *Diabetologia* 49 (5):1117–1119. doi: 10.1007/s00125-006-0196-5.

Benyshek, Daniel C., John F. Martin, and Carol S. Johnston. 2001. "A reconsideration of the origins of the type 2 diabetes epidemic among native Americans and the implications for intervention policy." *Medical Anthropology* 20 (1):25–64. doi: 10.1080/01459740.2001.9966186.

Bermudez, Odilia I, and Katherine L. Tucker. 2003. "Trends in dietary patterns of Latin American populations." *Cadernos de Saúde Pública* 19:S87–S99.

Bernard, Russell H. 2006. *Research Methods in Anthropology, Fourth Edition, Qualitative and Quantitative Approaches*. Lanham: Altamira Press.

Beyene, Yewoubdar. 1986. "Cultural significance and physiological manifestations of menopause a biocultural analysis." *Culture, Medicine and Psychiatry* 10 (1):47–71.

Blakely, Michael L. 1998. "Beyond European enlightenment: Toward a critical and humanistic human biology." In *Building a New Biocultural Synthesis: Political-Economic Perspectives on Human Biology*, edited by Alan H. and Thomas L. Leatherman Goodman, 379–406. Ann Arbor: University of Michigan Press.

Bleasdale, Sue. 2006. "Connecting paradise, culture and tourism in Tunisia." *Journal of Intercultural Studies* 27 (4):447–460.

Bogin, Barry. 1995. "Plasticity in the growth of Mayan refugee children living in the United States." In *Human Variability and Plasticity*, edited by C.G.N. Mascie-Taylor and Barry Bogin. New York: Cambridge University Press.

Bogin, Barry, and Holly B. Smith. 2012. "Evolution of the human life cycle." In *Human Biology: An Evolutionary and Biocultural Perspective*, edited by Sara Stinson, Barry Bogin, and Dennis O'Rourke. Hoboken: John Wiley & Sons.

Bolabola, Cema. 1981. "Does tourism cause malnutrition? They seem to be connected." *Pacific Perspective* 10 (1):72–77.

Borders, Ann E. Bryant, William A. Grobman, Laura B. Amsden, and Jane L. Holl. 2007. "Chronic stress and low birth weight neonates in a low-income population of women." *Obstetrics & Gynecology* 109 (2, Part 1):331–338.

Borofsky, Robert. 2002. "The four subfields: Anthropologists as mythmakers." *American Anthropologist* 104 (2):463–480.

Bosu, William K. 2015. "An overview of the nutrition transition in West Africa: Implications for non-communicable diseases." *Proceedings of the nutrition society* 74 (4):466–477.

Bourdieu, Pierre. 1977. *Outline of a Theory of Practice*. Translated by R. Nice. Cambridge" Cambridge University Press.

Brewis, Alexandra. 2003. "Biocultural aspects of obesity in young Mexican schoolchildren." *American Journal of Human Biology* 15 (3):446–460.

Browner, Carole H. 1989. "Women, household and health in Latin America." *Social Science & Medicine* 28 (5):461–473.

Bruijnzeel, L. A., L. S. Hamilton, and F. N. Scatena. 2010. *Tropical Montane Cloud Forests [Electronic Resource]: Science for Conservation and Management, International Hydrology Series*. Leiden: Cambridge University Press, 2010.

Caballero, Jose Maria. 1984. "Agriculture and the peasantry under industrialization pressures: Lessons from the Peruvian experience." *Latin American Research Review* 19 (2):3–41.

Cantor, Allison, Charlotte Noble, Adrian Seal-Feldman, Cattie Trucksess, and Dawn Waltonbaugh. 2008. "'De Donde Viene Su Comida?' Participación en la Feri a de Agricultor." In *Community Health 2008*. Monteverde: University of South Florida and the Monteverde Institute.

Cantor, Allison, Jenny Peña, and David Himmelgreen. 2013. "'We Never Ate Like That, Not Fast Food, or Junk Foods': Accounts of changing maternal diet in a

Tourist Community in Rural Costa Rica." *Ecology of Food and Nutrition* 52 (6):479–496.

Cantor, Allison R., Isabella Chan, and Kristina Baines. 2018. "From the Chacra to the Tienda: Dietary delocalization in the Peruvian Andes." *Food and Foodways* 26 (3):198–222.

Carey, James W. 1990. "Social system effects on local level morbidity and adaptation in the rural Peruvian Andes." *Medical Anthropology Quarterly* 4 (3):266–295. doi: 10.1525/maq.1990.4.3.02a00020.

Carmichael, Suzan L., Wei Yang, Amy Herring, Barbara Abrams, and Gary M. Shaw. 2007. "Maternal food insecurity is associated with increased risk of certain birth defects." *The Journal of Nutrition* 137 (9):2087–2092.

Castillo, V. Oscar, Francisco Mardones S., and Jaime Rozowski N. 2011. "Patrones alimentarios en embarazadas de bajo peso de la región metropolitana." *Revista chilena de nutrición* 38 (2):117–126. doi: 10.4067/s0717-75182011000200002.

CCSA. 2018. "National system of conservation areas." http://www.costarica-nationalparks.com/.

Chavez, Adolfo, Celia Martínez, and Beatriz Soberanes. 1995. "The effect of malnutrition on human development: A 24-year study of well-nourished and malnourished children living in a poor Mexican village." *Nutritional Anthropology: Biocultural Perspectives on Food and Nutrition* 234–252.

Choudhry, Ushvendra Kaur. 1997. "Traditional practices of women from India: Pregnancy, childbirth, and newborn care." *Journal of Obstetric, Gynecologic, & Neonatal Nursing* 26 (5):533–539.

Christian, Parul, Shipra Bunjun Srihari, Andrew Thorne-Lyman, Subarna K. Khatry, Steven C. LeClerq, and Sharada Ram Shrestha. 2006. "Eating down in pregnancy: Exploring food-related beliefs and practices of pregnancy in rural Nepal." *Ecology of Food and Nutrition* 45 (4):253–278.

Christians, Clifford G. 2011. "Ethics and politics in qualitative research." In *The SAGE Handbook of Qualitative Research*, edited by Norma K. Denzin and Yvonna S. Lincoln. Los Angeles: SAGE.

Coates, Jennfier, Swindale, Anne, and Paula Bilinsky. 2007. Household Food Insecurity Access Scale (HFIAS) for measurement of household food access: Indicator guide (v.3). In *Food and Nutrition Technical Assistance Project*. Washington, DC: Academy for Educational Development.

Coffey, Brian. 1993. "Investment incentives as a means of encouraging tourism development: The case of Costa Rica." *Bulletin of Latin American Research* 12 (1):83–90.

Coleman-Jensen, Alisha J. 2011. "Working for peanuts: Nonstandard work and food insecurity across household structure." *Journal of Family and Economic Issues* 32 (1):84–97.

Corman, Hope, Kelly Noonan, and Nancy E. Reichman. 2014. "Effects of infant health on family food insecurity: Evidence from two U.S. birth cohort studies." *Social Science & Medicine* 123:18–25. doi: http://dx.doi.org/10.1016/j.socscimed.2014.10.041.

Council, World Travel & Tourism. 2018. *Travel & Tourism Economic Impact 2018 Costa Rica*. Edited by Rochelle Turner. London: World Travel & Tourism Council.

Cowherd, Robert Eugene. 2012. "The effects of food insecurity on mental wellbeing in Monteverde Costa Rica." Master of Arts, Department of Anthropology, University of South Florida.

Creedman, Theodore S. 1991. *Costa Rica*. Vol. 16. Scarecrow Press.

Crump, Martha L., Frank R. Hensley, and Kenneth L. Clark. 1992. "Apparent decline of the golden toad: Underground or extinct?" *Copeia* 413–420.

Cukier, Judie, Joanne Norris, and Geoffrey Wall. 1996. "The involvement of women in the tourism industry of Bali, Indonesia." *The Journal of Development Studies* 33 (2):248–270.

Daltabuit, Magalí, and Thomas L. Leatherman. 1998. "The biocultural impact of tourism on Mayan communities." In *Building a New Biocultural Synthesis: Political-Economic Perspectives on Human Biology*, edited by Alan H. Goodman and Thomas L. Leatherman, 317–338. Ann Arbor: University of Michigan Press.

Dalzell, S.E., L.M.A. Jarjou, A. Prentice, K. Ward, and G.R. Goldberg. 2017. "Dietary intakes of Gambian women: Impact of the nutrition transition." *Proceedings of the Nutrition Society* 76 (OCE4).

Damschroder, Laura J., David C. Aron, Rosalind E. Keith, Susan R. Kirsh, Jeffery A. Alexander, and Julie C. Lowery. 2009. "Fostering implementation of health services research findings into practice: A consolidated framework for advancing implementation science." *Implement Science* 4 (1):50.

Dancause, Kelsey N., Miguel Vilar, Chim Chan, Christa DeHuff, Michelle Wilson, Laura E. Soloway, Len Tarivonda, Ralph Regenvanu, Akira Kaneko, and Ralph M. Garruto. 2012. "Patterns of childhood and adolescent overweight and obesity during health transition in Vanuatu." *Public Health Nutrition* 15 (1):158–166.

de la Torre, Adela, and Lynda Rush. 1987. "The determinants of breastfeeding for Mexican migrant women." *International Migration Review* 728–742.

Delormier, Treena, Katherine L. Frohlich, and Louise Potvin. 2009. "Food and eating as social practice–understanding eating patterns as social phenomena and implications for public health." *Sociology of Health & Illness* 31 (2):215–228.

D'Epiro, JoHanna, Aaron Lampkin, Loralee Trocio, and Jaime Wilke. 2002. Acce so al Servicio de Atención Prenatal para las Mujeres de la Zona de Monteverde hasta el Momento del Parto. In *Community Health 2002*. Monteverde: University of South Florida and the Monteverde Institute.

del Rocío Sáenz, María, Juan Luis Bermúdez, and Mónica Acosta. 2011. "Universal coverage in a middle income country: Costa Rica." *World Health Report (2010) Background Paper, No. 11,* Geneva: World Health Organization.

Dewey, Kathryn G. 1989. "Nutrition and the commoditization of food systems in Latin America and the Caribbean." *Social Science & Medicine* 28 (5):415–424.

Dewing, Sarah, Mark Tomlinson, Ingrid M. Le Roux, Mickey Chopra, and Alexander C. Tsai. 2013. "Food insecurity and its association with co-occurring postnatal depression, hazardous drinking, and suicidality among women in peri-urban South Africa." *Journal of Affective Disorders* 150 (2):460–465.

Dodd, Warren. 2011. "Towards a political ecology of nutritional transitions in Central America: The construction of nutrient-deficient ecologies." *Totem: The University of Western Ontario Journal of Anthropology* 19 (1):10.

Dolatian, Mahrokh, Nasibeh Sharifi, and Zohreh Mahmoodi. 2018. "Relationship of socioeconomic status, psychosocial factors, and food insecurity with preterm labor: A longitudinal study." *International Journal of Reproductive Biomedicine* 16 (9):563.

Drewnowski, A. 2009. "Obesity, diets, and social inequalities." *Nutrition Reviews* 67 (5):S36–S39. doi: 10.1111/j.1753-4887.2009.00157.x.

Drewnowski, Adam, Anju Aggarwal, Philip M. Hurvitz, Pablo Monsivais, and Anne V. Moudon. 2012. "Obesity and supermarket access: Proximity or price?" *American Journal of Public Health* 102 (8):e74–e80.

Drewnowski, Adam, and Barry M. Popkin. 1997. "The nutrition transition: New trends in the global diet." *Nutrition Reviews* 55 (2):31–43. doi: 10.1111/j.1753-4887.1997.tb01593.x.

Dufour, Darna L., and Richard L. Bender. 2013. "Nutrition transitions: A view from anthropology." In *Nutritional Anthropology: Biocultural Perspectives on Food and Nutrition, Second Edition*, edited by Darna L. Dufour, Alan H. Goodman, and Gretel H. Pelto, 372–382. Oxford: Oxford University Press.

Durkheim, Emile. 1982. *Rules of Sociological Method.* Simon and Schuster.

ENAHO. 2018. *Encuesta Nacional de Hogares: Resultados Generales*, año 7. San José, Costa Rica: Instituto Nacional de Estadística y Censos.

Facchinetti, F., G. Pedrielli, G. Benoni, M. Joppi, G. Verlato, G. Dante, S. Balduzzi, and L. Cuzzolin. 2012. "Herbal supplements in pregnancy: Unexpected results from a multicentre study." *Human Reproduction* 27 (11):3161–3167.

Farmer, Paul. 2001. *Infections and Inequalities: The Modern Plagues*. University of California Press.

Farmer, Paul. 2005. *Pathologies of Power: Health, Human Rights, and the New War on the Poor: With a New Preface by the Author*. Vol. 4. University of California Press.

Feinsinger, P. 1976. "Organization of a tropical guild of Nectarivorous birds." *Ecological Monographs* 46 (3):257–291. doi: 10.2307/1942255.

Ferguson, Lucy. 2010. "Tourism development and the restructuring of social reproduction in Central America." *Review of International Political Economy* 17 (5):860–888.

Ferguson, Lucy. 2011. "Promoting gender equality and empowering women? Tourism and the third millennium development goal." *Current Issues in Tourism* 14 (3):235–249. doi: 10.1080/13683500.2011.555522.

Ferzacca, Steve. 2012. "Diabetes and culture." *Annual Review of Anthropology* 41:411–426.

Field, Andy. 2009. *Discovering Statistics using SPSS*. Sage Publications.

Filozof, C., C. Gonzalez, M. Sereday, C. Mazza, and J. Braguinsky. 2001. "Obesity prevalence and trends in Latin-American countries." *Obesity Reviews,* 2 (2):99–106.

Fisberg, Mauro, Irina Kovalskys, Georgina Gómez, Attilio Rigotti, Lilia Sanabria, Martha García, Rossina Torres, Marianella Herrera-Cuenca, Ioná Zimberg, and Berthold Koletzko. 2018. "Total and added sugar intake: Assessment in eight Latin American countries." *Nutrients* 10 (4):389.

Fischer, Nils C., Teresa Shamah-Levy, Verónica Mundo-Rosas, Ignacio Méndez-Gómez-Humarán, and Rafael Pérez-Escamilla. 2014. "Household food insecurity is associated with anemia in adult Mexican women of reproductive age." *The Journal of Nutrition* 144 (12):2066–2072.

Fisher, David. 2004. "The demonstration effect revisited." *Annals of Tourism Research* 31 (2):428–446.

Fouts, Hillary N., Barry S. Hewlett, and Michael E. Lamb. 2012. "A biocultural approach to breastfeeding interactions in central Africa." *American Anthropologist* 114 (1):123–136.

Franklin, Brandi, Ashley Jones, Dejuan Love, Stephane Puckett, Justin Macklin, and Shelley White-Means. 2012. "Exploring mediators of food insecurity and obesity: A review of recent literature." *Journal of Community Health* 37 (1):253–264.

Friel, Sharon, Deborah Gleeson, Anne-Marie Thow, Ronald Labonte, David Stuckler, Adrian Kay, and Wendy Snowdon. 2013. "A new generation of trade policy: Potential risks to diet-related health from the trans pacific partnership agreement." *Globalization and Health* 9 (1):1.

Frith, Amy L., Ruchira T. Naved, Lars Ake Persson, Kathleen M. Rasmussen, and Edward A. Frongillo. 2012. "Early participation in a prenatal food supplementation program ameliorates the negative association of food insecurity with quality of maternal-infant interaction." *The Journal of Nutrition* 142 (6):1095–1101.

Frohlick, Susan. 2013. "Intimate tourism markets: Money, gender, and the complexity of erotic exchange in a Costa Rican Caribbean Town." *Mercados de Turismo Íntimo: Dinero, Género, y la Complej idad del Intercambio Erótico en un pueblo caribeño de Costa Rica.* 86 (1):133–162.

Frohlick, Susan. 2016. "Feeling sexual transgression: Subjectivity, bodily experience, and non-normative hetero-erotic practices in women's cross-border sex in Costa Rica." *Gender, Place & Culture* 23 (2):257–273.

Fuhrmann, Hollie, Jennifer Garcia, Nicole Haykin, Rebecca Sameroff, and Rebecca Todd. 2006. "De eso no se habla": An explorative study on the sexual and reproductive health education of adolescents in the Monteverde Zone. In *Community Health 2006*. Monteverde: University of South Florida and the Monteverde Institute.

Gebremedhin, Samson, Fikre Enquselassie, and Melaku Umeta. 2011. "Prevalence of prenatal zinc deficiency and its association with socio-demographic, dietary and health care related factors in Rural Sidama, Southern Ethiopia: A cross-sectional study." *BMC public health* 11 (1):898.

Gentry, Kristine McKenzie. 2007. "Belizean women and tourism work: Opportunity or impediment?" *Annals of Tourism Research* 34 (2):477–496. doi: http://dx.doi.org/10.1016/j.annals.2006.11.003.

Giddens, Anthony. 1979. *Central Problems in Social Theory: Action, Structure and Contradictions in Social Analysis*. Vol. 241: University of California Press.

Gindling, T.H., and Juan Diego Trejos. 2005. "Accounting for changing earnings inequality in Costa Rica, 1980–99." *Journal of Development Studies* 41 (5):898–926.

Giordano, C., and D.C. Benyshek. 2015. "DOHaD research with populations in transition: A case study of prenatal diet remote recall with Yup'ik Alaskan women." *Journal of Developmental Origins of Health and Disease* 6 (2):79–87.

Glover, Vivette. 2014. "Maternal depression, anxiety and stress during pregnancy and child outcome; what needs to be done." *Best Practice & Research Clinical Obstetrics & Gynaecology* 28 (1):25–35.

Gluckman, Peter, and Mark Hanson, eds. 2006. *The Developmental Origins of Health and Disease*. Cambridge: Cambridge University Press.

Gluckman, P. D., and M. A. Hanson. 2008. "Developmental and epigenetic pathways to obesity: An evolutionary-developmental perspective." *International Journal of Obesity* 32:S62–S71. doi: 10.1038/ijo.2008.240.

Godfrey, Keith. 2006. "The 'developmental origins' hypothesis: Epidemiology." In *Developmental Origins of Health and Disease*, edited by Peter Gluckman and Mark Hanson, 6–33. United Kingdom: Cambridge University Press.

Goffman, Erving. 1959. *The Presentation of Self in Everyday Life*. New York: Anchor Books/Doubleday, 1959.

Goffman, Erving. 1967. *Interaction Ritual; Essays on Face-to-Face Behavior, Anchor Books: A596*: Garden City, NY: Doubleday, 1967.

Goodman, Alan H., and Thomas L. Leatherman. 1998. *Building a New Biocultural Synthesis: Political-Economic Perspectives on Human Biology*. University of Michigan Press.

Goodman, Alan H., and Thomas L. Leatherman. 1998. "Traversing the chasm between biology and culture: An introduction." *Building a New Biocultural Synthesis: Political-Economic Perspectives on Human Biology*, 3–42.

Gross, Rachel S., Alan L. Mendelsohn, and Mary Jo Messito. 2018. "Additive effects of household food insecurity during pregnancy and infancy on maternal infant feeding styles and practices." *Appetite* 130:20–28.

Gustafson, David, Alona Gutman, Whitney Leet, Adam Drewnowski, Jessica Fanzo, and John Ingram. 2016. "Seven food system metrics of sustainable nutrition security." *Sustainability* 8 (3):196.

Hamilton, Debra. 2015. "Number of Tourists."

Hamilton, Lawrence S., James O. Juvik, and Fred N. Scatena. 1995. "The Puerto Rico tropical cloud forest symposium: Introduction and workshop synthesis." In *Tropical Montane Cloud Forests*, 1–18. Springer.

Hamm, Thomas D. 2004. *The Quakers in America. [electronic resource], Columbia Contemporary American Religion Series*. New York: Columbia University Press, 2004.

Hammer, Patricia J., Carmen Monasterios, and Kiyomi Tsuyuki. 2004. *Guía de autodiagnóstico comunitario de Investigación participativa comunitaria de las necesidades frente a problemas en la 1ra mitad del embarazo. Manual para facilitadores*. Bolivia: Programa PAC Bolivia.

Handler, Richard. 2012. "What's up, Doctor Goffman? Tell us where the action is!" *Journal of the Royal Anthropological Institute* 18 (1):179–190. doi: 10.1111/j.1467-9655.2011.01737.x.

Hanson, M.A., and P.D. Gluckman. 2015. "Developmental origins of health and disease–global public health implications." *Best Practice & Research Clinical Obstetrics & Gynaecology* 29 (1):24–31.

Hartini, T. Ninuk S., R. Siwi Padmawati, Lars Lindholm, Achmad, Surjono, Anna Winkvist. 2005. "The importance of eating rice: Changing food habits among pregnant Indonesian women during the economic crisis." *Social Science & Medicine* 61:199–210. doi: 10.1016/j.socscimed.2004.11.043.

Hawkes, Corinna. 2006. "Uneven dietary development: Linking the policies and processes of globalization with the nutrition transition, obesity and diet-related chronic diseases." *Globalization and Health* 2 (1):4.

Hawkes, Corinna. 2008. "Dietary implications of supermarket development: A global perspective." *Development Policy Review* 26 (6):657–692. doi: 10.1111/j.1467-7679.2008.00428.x.

Hawkes, Corinna, and Anne Marie Thow. 2008. "Implications of the Central America-Dominican Republic-Free Trade Agreement for the nutrition transition in Central America." *Revista Panamericana de Salud Pública* 24 (5):345–360.

Hawks, Steven R., Ray M. Merrill, Hala N. Madanat, Takeo Miyagawa, Jiraporn Suwanteerangkul, Cipriano M. Guarin, and Chen Shaofang. 2004. "Intuitive eating and the nutrition transition in Asia." *Asia Pacific Journal of Clinical Nutrition* 13 (2):194–203.

Henrich, Joseph, and Natalie Henrich. 2010. "The evolution of cultural adaptations: Fijian food taboos protect against dangerous marine toxins." *Proceedings of the Royal Society of London B: Biological Sciences* 277 (1701):3715–3724.

Hicks, Raymond, Helen V. Milner, and Dustin Tingley. 2014. "Trade policy, economic interests, and party politics in a developing country: The political economy of CAFTA-DR." *International Studies Quarterly* 58 (1):106–117.

Himmelgreen, David, A. Romero-Daza, NancyEdgar Amador, and Cynthia Pace. 2013. "Tourism, economic insecurity, and nutritional health in Rural Costa Rica: Using Syndemic theory to understand the impacts of the globalizing economy at the local level."

Himmelgreen, David, Nancy Romero-Daza, Allison Cantor, and Sara Arias. 2014. "Is the cup half empty or half full? Economic transition and changing ideas about food insecurity in Rural Costa Rica." In *Women Redefining the Experience of Food Insecurity: Life off the Edge of the Table*, edited by Janet Page-Reeves. Lexington Books.

Himmelgreen, David A., Nancy Romero Daza, Maribel Vega, Humberto Brenes Cambronero, and Edgar Amador. 2006. "'The Tourist Season Goes Down But Not the Prices.' Tourism and food insecurity in rural Costa Rica." *Ecology of Food and Nutrition* 45 (4):295–321.

Honey, Martha. 2008. *Ecotourism and Sustainable Development: Who Owns Paradise?* Island Press.

Horton, Lynn R. 2009. "Buying up nature: Economic and social impacts of Costa Rica's ecotourism boom." *Latin American Perspectives* 36 (3):93–107. doi: 10.1177/0094582x09334299.

Hrdy, Sarah Blaffer. 2009. *Mothers and Others*. Harvard UP: Cambridge, MA.

Hromi-Fiedler, Amber, Angela Bermúdez-Millán, Sofia Segura-Pérez, and Rafael Pérez-Escamilla. 2011. "Household food insecurity is associated with depressive symptoms among low-income pregnant Latinas." *Maternal & Child Nutrition* 7 (4):421–430.

Hunt, Carter A., William H. Durham, Laura Driscoll, and Martha Honey. 2015. "Can ecotourism deliver real economic, social, and environmental benefits? A study of the Osa Peninsula, Costa Rica." *Journal of Sustainable Tourism* 23 (3):339–357.

Hvalkof, Soren, and Arturo Escobar. 1998. "Nature, political ecology, and social practice: Toward an academic and political agenda " In *Building a New Biocultural Synthesis: Political-Economic Perspectives on Human Biology*, edited by Alan H. and Thomas L. Leatherman Goodman, 425–450. Ann Arbor: University of Michigan Press.

Ice, Gilliam, and Gary D. James. 2012. "Stress and human biology." In *Human Biology: An Evolutionary and Biocultural Perspective, Second Edition*, edited by Barry Bogin and Dennis O'Rourke Sara Stinson. Hoboken: John Wiley & Sons, Inc.

ICT. 2017. *Divisas por concepto de turismo*. Instituto Costarricense de Turismo Planeamiento y Desarrollo Turístico Administración de la Información.

ICT. 2018. "Empleo en las actividades asociadas con el sector turístico." In *Metadatos de los Indicadores*. Instituto Costarricense de Turismo: Dirección de Planeamiento y Desarrollo Turístico Unidad de Administración de la Información.

Incorporated, Cargill. 2015. "Cargill en Costa Rica." http://www.cargill.com.hn/es/nosotros-en-centroamerica/costa-rica/index.jsp.

INEC. 2011. "Población total por sexo según provincia, cantón y distrito, censo 2011." INEC. http://datos.inec.go.cr/datastreams/74800/poblacion-total-por-sexo-segun-provincia-canton-y-distrito-censo-2011/.

Ivers, Louise C., and Kimberly A. Cullen. 2011. "Food insecurity: Special considerations for women." *The American Journal of Clinical Nutrition* 94 (6):1740S–1744S.

Izugbara, C. Otutubikey. 2003. "The cultural context of geophagy among pregnant and lactating Ngwa women of Southeastern Nigeria." *African Anthropologist* 10 (2):180–199.

Jaacks, Lindsay M., Justine Kavle, Abigail Perry, and Albertha Nyaku. 2017. "Programming maternal and child overweight and obesity in the context of undernutrition: Current evidence and key considerations for low-and middle-income countries." *Public Health Nutrition* 20 (7):1286–1296.

Jayawardena, Ranil, Priyanga Ranasinghe, Maheshi Wijayabandara, Andrew P. Hills, and Anoop Misra. 2017. "Nutrition transition and obesity among teenagers and young adults in South Asia." *Current Diabetes Reviews* 13 (5):444–451.

Jebena, Mulusew G., Mohammed Taha, Motohiro Nakajima, Andrine Lemieux, Fikre Lemessa, Richard Hoffman, Markos Tesfaye, Tefera Belachew, Netsanet Workineh, and Esayas Kebede. 2015. "Household food insecurity and mental distress among pregnant women in Southwestern Ethiopia: A cross sectional study design." *BMC Pregnancy and Childbirth* 15 (1):250.

Johns, Timothy, and Lindi Sibeko. 2003. "Pregnancy outcomes in women using herbal therapies." *Birth Defects Research Part B: Developmental and Reproductive Toxicology* 68 (6):501–504.

Junges, Carolina Frescura, Lúcia Beatriz Ressel, and Marisa Monticelli. 2014. "Amongst wishes and possibilities: Eating habits of pregnant women from an urban community in Southern Brazil." *Texto & Contexto-Enfermagem* 23 (2):382–390.

Kain, Juliana, Fernando Vio, and Cecilia Albala. 2003. "Obesity trends and determinant factors in Latin America." *Cadernos de Saúde Pública* 19:S77–S86.

Kavle, Justine A, Sohair Mehanna, Ghada Khan, Mohamed Hassan, Gulsen Saleh, and Cyril Engmann. 2018. "Program considerations for integration of nutrition and family planning: Beliefs around maternal diet and breastfeeding within the context of the nutrition transition in Egypt." *Maternal & Child Nutrition* 14 (1):e12469.

Kaye, Kerwin. 2012. "De-medicalizing addiction: Toward biocultural understandings." In *Critical Perspectives on Addiction,* edited by Julie Netherland. London: Emerald Group Publishing Limited, 27–51.

Key, Carol Jane. 2002. "The political economy of the transition from fishing to tourism, in Placencia, Belize." *International Review of Modern Sociology* 30 (1/2) 1–18.

Kirtsoglou, Elisabeth, and Dimitrios Theodossopoulos. 2004. "'They are taking our culture away' tourism and culture commodification in the Garifuna Community of Roatan." *Critique of Anthropology* 24 (2):135–157.

Kleiser, Christina, Gert Mensink, Hannelore Neuhauser, Liane Schenk, and Bärbel-Maria Kurth. 2010. "Food intake of young people with a migration background living in Germany." *Public Health Nutrition* 13 (03):324–330.

Knauft, Bruce M. 1996. "Genealogies for the present in cultural anthropology." Londong: Routledge.

Koehler-Geib, Friederike, and Susana M. Sanchez. 2015. *Costa Rica Five Years After CAFTA-DR: Assessing Early Results.* The World Bank.

Koeppel, Dan. 2007. *Banana: The Fate of the Fruit that Changed the World.* Penguin.

Kovalskys, Irina, Mauro Fisberg, Georgina Gómez, Rossina G. Pareja, Martha C. Yépez García, Lilia Y. Cortés Sanabria, Marianella Herrera-Cuenca, Attilio Rigotti, Viviana Guajardo, and Ioná Zalcman Zimberg. 2018. "Energy intake and food sources of eight Latin American countries: Results from the Latin American Study of Nutrition and Health (ELANS)." *Public Health Nutrition* 21 (14):2535–2547.

Kuzawa, Christopher W., and Elizabeth A. Quinn. 2009. "Developmental origins of adult function and health: Evolutionary hypotheses." *Annual Review of Anthropology* 38 (1):131–147. doi: doi:10.1146/annurev-anthro-091908-164350.

Laderman, Carol. 1987. "Destructive heat and cooling prayer: Malay humoralism in pregnancy, childbirth and the postpartum period." *Social Science & Medicine* 25 (4):357–365. doi: http://dx.doi.org/10.1016/0277-9536(87)90274-7.

Lang, Hartmut, Peter Challenor, and Peter D. Killworth. 2004. "A new addition to the family of space sampling methods." *Field Methods* 16 (1):55–69.

Laraia, Barbara, Lisa C. Vinikoor-Imler, and Anna Maria Siega-Riz. 2015. "Food insecurity during pregnancy leads to stress, disordered eating, and greater postpartum weight among overweight women." *Obesity* 23 (6):1303–1311.

Laraia, Barbara A., Anna Maria Siega-Riz, and Craig Gundersen. 2010. "Household food insecurity is associated with self-reported pregravid weight status, gestational weight gain, and pregnancy complications." *Journal of the American Dietetic Association* 110 (5):692–701.

Laraia, Barbara A., Anna Maria Siega-Riz, Craig Gundersen, and Nancy Dole. 2006. "Psychosocial factors and socioeconomic indicators are associated with household food insecurity among pregnant women." *The Journal of nutrition* 136 (1):177–182.

Lau, Christopher, John M. Rogers, Mina Desai, and Michael G. Ross. 2011. "Fetal programming of adult disease: Implications for prenatal care." *Obstetrics & Gynecology* 117 (4):978–985.

Leatherman, Tom, and Alan H. Goodman. 2011. "Critical biocultural approaches in medical anthropology." In *A Companion to Medical Anthropology*, edited by Merrill Singer and Pamela I. Anderson, 29–47. West Sussex: Wiley-Blackwell.

Leatherman, Thomas L. 1996. "A biocultural perspective on health and household economy in southern Peru." *Medical Anthropology Quarterly* 10 (4):476–495.

Leatherman, Thomas L., Alan H. Goodman, and Tobias Stillman. 2010. "Changes in stature, weight, and nutritional status with tourism-based economic development in the Yucatan." *Economics & Human Biology* 8 (2):153–158. doi: http://dx.doi.org/10.1016/j.ehb.2010.05.008.

Leatherman, Thomas L., and Alan Goodman. 2005. "Coca-colonization of diets in the Yucatan." *Social Science and Medicine* 61 (4):833–846.

Lee, Dominic T.S., Iris S.L. Ngai, Mandy M.T. Ng, Ingrid H. Lok, Alexander S.K. Yip, and Tony K.H. Chung. 2009. "Antenatal taboos among Chinese women in Hong Kong." *Midwifery* 25 (2):104–113.

Legislativa, Asamblea. 1943. *Código de Trabajo de Costa Rica.* Asamblea Legislativa de Costa Rica.

Lende, Daniel H. 2005. "Wanting and drug use: A biocultural approach to the analysis of addiction." *Ethos* 33 (1):100–124.

Lende, Daniel H. 2012. "Poverty poisons the brain." *Annals of Anthropological Practice* 36 (1):183–201.

Levins, Richard, and Richard C. Lewontin. 1985. *The Dialectical Biologist.* Harvard University Press.

Levins, Richard, and Richard Lewontin. 1998. "Foreword." In *Building a New Biocultural Synthesis: Political-Economic Perspective on Human Biology*, edited by Alan H. and Thomas L. Leatherman Goodman, x–xv. Ann Arbor: University of Michigan Press.

Li, Shu-Chen. 2003. "Biocultural orchestration of developmental plasticity across levels: The interplay of biology and culture in shaping the mind and behavior across the life span." *Psychological Bulletin* 129 (2):171.

Littleton, Heather L., Kimberly Bye, Katie Buck, and Amanda Amacker. 2010. "Psychosocial stress during pregnancy and perinatal outcomes: A meta-analytic review." *Journal of Psychosomatic Obstetrics & Gynecology* 31 (4):219–228.

Livingstone, Frank B. 1958. "Anthropological implications of sickle cell gene distribution in West Africa." *American Anthropologist* 60 (3):533–562.

Lundgren, Nancy. 1993. "Women, work and 'Development' in Belize." *Dialectical Anthropology* 18 (3/4):363–378. doi: 10.2307/29790543.

Machín, Leandro, Ana Giménez, Leticia Vidal, and Gastón Ares. 2014. "Influence of context on motives underlying food choice." *Journal of Sensory Studies* 29 (5):313–324.

Mak, Athena H.N., Margaret Lumbers, and Anita Eves. 2012. "Globalisation and food consumption in tourism." *Annals of Tourism Research* 39 (1):171–196.

Martínez, Gustavo J. 2008. "Traditional practices, beliefs and uses of medicinal plants in relation to maternal–baby health of Criollo woman in central Argentina." *Midwifery* 24 (4):490–502. doi: http://dx.doi.org/10.1016/j.midw.2006.12.011.

Martínez, Rodrigo, Amalia Palma, Eduardo Atalah, and Anna Christina Pinheiro. 2009. "Food and nutrition insecurity in Latin America and the Caribbean." *United*

Nations, World Food Programme. Economic Commission for Latin America (ECLAC).

Martorell, Reynaldo, and Amanda Zongrone. 2012. "Intergenerational influences on child growth and undernutrition." *Paediatric and Perinatal Epidemiology* 26 (s1):302–314.

Martorell, Reynaldo, Laura Kettel Khan, Morgen L. Hughes, and Laurence M. Grummer-Strawn. 1998. "Obesity in Latin American women and children." *The Journal of Nutrition* 128 (9):1464–1473.

Maxwell, Simon. 1998. "Saucy with the Gods: Nutrition and food security speak to poverty." *Food Policy* 23 (3):215–230.

McDade, Thomas. 2005. "Life history, maintenance, and the early origins of immune function." *American Journal of Human Biology* 17 (1):81–94.

McDade, Thomas W. 2002. "Status incongruity in Samoan youth: A biocultural analysis of culture change, stress, and immune function." *Medical Anthropology Quarterly* 16 (2):123–150. doi: 10.2307/649486.

McIntyre, Lynn, N. Theresa Glanville, Kim D. Raine, Jutta B. Dayle, Bonnie Anderson, and Noreen Battaglia. 2003. "Do low-income lone mothers compromise their nutrition to feed their children?" *Canadian Medical Association Journal* 168 (6):686–691.

Melby, Melissa K., and Michelle Lampl. 2011. "Menopause, a biocultural perspective." *Annual Review of Anthropology* 40:53–70.

Melgar-Quinonez, Hugo, and Michelle Hackett. 2008. "Measuring household food security: The global experience." *Revista de Nutrição* 21:27s–37s.

Messer, Ellen. 1981. "Hot-cold classification: Theoretical and practical implications of a Mexican study." *Social Science & Medicine. Part B: Medical Anthropology* 15 (2):133–145.

Moffat, Tina. 2001. "A biocultural investigation of the Weanling's dilemma in Kathmandu, Nepal: Do universal recommendations for weaning practices make sense?" *Journal of Biosocial Science* 33 (3):321–338.

Molina, Iván, and Steven Palmer, eds. 2006. *The Costa Rica Reader: History, Culture Politics*. Durham: Duke University Press.

Montero, David, Marcia Bodero, Guillermina Riveros, Lisette Lapierre, Aldo Gaggero, Roberto Mauricio Vidal, and Maricel Vidal. 2015. "Molecular epidemiology and genetic diversity of Listeria monocytogenes isolates from a wide variety of ready-to-eat foods and their relationship to clinical strains from listeriosis outbreaks in Chile." *Frontiers in Microbiology* 6. doi: 10.3389/fmicb.2015.00384.

Monteverdeinfo. 2011. "Monteverde to Arenal Volcano." monteverdeinfo.com. http://www.monteverdeinfo.com/volcano.htm.

Moore, Latetia V., Ana V. Diez Roux, Jennifer A. Nettleton, and David R. Jacobs. 2008. "Associations of the local food environment with diet quality—A comparison of assessments based on surveys and geographic information systems the multi-ethnic study of atherosclerosis." *American Journal of Epidemiology* 167 (8):917–924.

Morgan, Lynn M. 1990. "International politics and primary health care in Costa Rica." *Social Science & Medicine* 30 (2):211–219. doi: http://dx.doi.org/10.1016/0277-9536(90)90082-4.

Morgan, Lynn M. 1998. "Latin American social medicine and the politics of theory." In *Building a New Biocultural Synthesis: Political-Economic Perspectives on Human Biology*, edited by Alan H. and Thomas L. Leatherman Goodman, 407–424. Ann Arbor: University of Michigan Press.

Morland, Kimberly, Ana V. Diez Roux, and Steve Wing. 2006. "Supermarkets, other food stores, and obesity: The atherosclerosis risk in communities study." *American Journal of Preventive Medicine* 30 (4):333–339.

Muller, Jocelyn, and Astier M. Almedom. 2008. "What is 'famine food'? Distinguishing between traditional vegetables and special foods for times of hunger/scarcity (Boumba, Niger)." *Human Ecology* 36 (4):599–607.

Myers, David N., Margarita Hill, and Stacy Anne Harwood. 2005. "Cross-cultural learning and study abroad: Transforming pedagogical outcomes." *Landscape Journal* 24 (2):172–184.

Nagata, Jason M., Frances K. Barg, Claudia R. Valeggia, and Kent D. W. Bream. 2011. "Coca-colonization and hybridization of diets among the Tz'utujil Maya." *Ecology of Food and Nutrition* 50 (4):297–318. doi: 10.1080/03670244.2011.568911.

Nakamura, Harunobu, Katsuyasu Kouda, WenYing Fan, and Hiroichi Takeuchi. 2002. "Cardiovascular risk factors in a tourist town: Association with job-related factors." *Journal of Physiological Anthropology and Applied Human Science* 21 (5):223–227.

Namey, Emily, Greg Guest, Lucy Thairu, and Laura Johnson. 2008. "Data reduction techniques for large qualitative data sets." *Handbook for Team-Based Qualitative Research*, 137–161.

Nebel, Sabine, Andrea Pieroni, and Michael Heinrich. 2006. "Ta chòrta: Wild edible greens used in the Graecanic area in Calabria, Southern Italy." *Appetite* 47 (3):333–342. doi: http://dx.doi.org/10.1016/j.appet.2006.05.010.

Nieto, F. Javier. 2015. "Siesta by decree or sound policy to promote sleep health? Lessons from a municipal proclamation in a rural Spanish town." *Sleep Health: Journal of the National Sleep Foundation* 1 (4):227–228.

NOAA. 2018. "What is a watershed?" National Ocean Service, National Oceanic and Atmospheric Administration, accessed March 23, 2019. https://oceanservice.noaa.gov/facts/watershed.html.

Obeyesekere, Gananath. 1963. "Pregnancy cravings (Dola-Duka) in relation to social structure and personality in a Sinhalese Village1." *American Anthropologist* 65 (2):323–342.

Oldewage-Theron, Wilna H., Emsie G. Dicks, and Carin E. Napier. 2006. "Poverty, household food insecurity and nutrition: Coping strategies in an informal settlement in the Vaal Triangle, South Africa." *Public Health* 120 (9):795–804. doi: http://dx.doi.org/10.1016/j.puhe.2006.02.009.

Olson, Christine M. 1999. "Nutrition and health outcomes associated with food insecurity and hunger." *The Journal of Nutrition* 129 (2):521S-524S.

Olson, Christine M, and Myla S Strawderman. 2008. "The relationship between food insecurity and obesity in rural childbearing women." *The Journal of Rural Health* 24 (1):60–66.

Omran, Abdel R. 1971. "The epidemiologic transition: A theory of the epidemiology of population change." *The Milbank Memorial Fund Quarterly* 49 (4):509–538. doi: 10.2307/3349375.

O'Neill, Alexander C. 2002. "What globalization means for ecotourism: Managing globalization's impacts on ecotourism in developing countries." *Indiana Journal of Global Legal Studies* 9 (2) 501–528.

Ono, M., A. Matsuyama, M. Karama, and S. Honda. 2013. "Association between social support and place of delivery: A cross-sectional study in Kericho, Western Kenya." *BMC Pregnancy and Childbirth* 13:9. doi: 10.1186/1471-2393-13-214.

Ortner, Sherry B. 1984. "Theory in Anthropology since the Sixties." *Comparative Studies in Society and History* 26 (1):126–166. doi: 10.2307/178524.

Ortner, Sherry B. 1997. *Making Gender: The Politics and Erotics of Culture*. Beacon Press.

Ortner, Sherry B. 2001. *Life and Death on Mt. Everest: Sherpas and Himalayan Mountaineering*. Princeton University Press.

Ortner, Sherry B. 2006. *Anthropology and Social Theory: Culture, Power, and the Acting Subject*. Duke University Press.

Otero, Gerardo, Gabriela Pechlaner, Giselle Liberman, and Efe Gürcan. 2015. "The neoliberal diet and inequality in the United States." *Social Science & Medicine* 142:47–55.

Oths, Kathryn S. 1998. "Assessing variation in health status in the Andes: A biocultural model." *Social Science & Medicine* 47 (8):1017–1030. doi: http://dx.doi.org/10.1016/S0277-9536(98)00161-0.

PAHO. 2015. "Country report: Costa Rica." Pan American Health Organization and the World Health Organization. https://www.paho.org/salud-en-las-americas-2017/?page_id=109.

PAHO. 2017. "Visualization of indicators for Costa Rica." Pan American Health Organization and the World Health Organization, accessed March 24 2019. http://www.paho.org/data/index.php/es/indicadores/visualizacion.html.

Painter, Rebecca C., Tessa J. Roseboom, and Otto P. Bleker. 2005. "Prenatal exposure to the Dutch famine and disease in later life: An overview." *Reproductive Toxicology* 20 (3):345–352. doi: http://dx.doi.org/10.1016/j.reprotox.2005.04.005.

Palmer, Iván Molina, and Steven. 2007. *Historia de Costa Rica*. San José: Universidad de Costa Rica.

Papan, Andrea S., and Barbara Clow. 2015. "The food insecurity——Obesity paradox as a vicious cycle for women: Inequalities and health." *Gender & Development* 23 (2):299–317.

Park, C. Y., and H. A. Eicher-Miller. 2014. "Iron deficiency is associated with food insecurity in pregnant females in the United States: National Health and Nutrition Examination Survey 1999–2010." *Journal of the Academy of Nutrition and Dietetics* 114 (12):1967–1973. doi: 10.1016/j.jand.2014.04.025.

Parra, Diana C., Lora Iannotti, Luis F. Gomez, Helena Pachón, Debra Haire-Joshu, Olga L. Sarmiento, Anne Sebert Kuhlmann, and Ross C. Brownson. 2015. "The nutrition transition in Colombia over a decade: A novel household classification system of anthropometric measures." *Archives of Public Health* 73 (1):12.

Perez-Escamilla, Rafael, Chessa Lutter, Ana Maria Segall, and Ada Rivera. 1995. "Exclusive breast-feeding duration is associated with attitudinal, socioeconomic and biocultural determinants in three Latin American countries." *The Journal of nutrition* 125 (12):2972.

Phillips, Wendy. 2005. "Cravings, marks, and open pores: Acculturation and preservation of pregnancy-related beliefs and practices among mothers of African descent in the United States." *Ethos* 33 (2) 231–255.

Piperata, Barbara Ann. 2008. "Forty days and forty nights: A biocultural perspective on postpartum practices in the Amazon." *Social Science & Medicine* 67 (7):1094–1103.

Piperata, Barbara A., Jennifer E. Spence, Pedro Da-Gloria, and Mark Hubbe. 2011. "The nutrition transition in Amazonia: Rapid economic change and its impact on growth and development in Ribeirinhos." *American Journal of Physical Anthropology* 146 (1):1–13.

Piperata, Barbara A., Kammi K. Schmeer, Craig Hadley, and Genevieve Ritchie-Ewing. 2013. "Dietary inequalities of mother–child pairs in the rural Amazon: Evidence of maternal-child buffering?" *Social Science & Medicine* 96:183–191. doi: http://dx.doi.org/10.1016/j.socscimed.2013.07.024.

Popkin, Barry. 2002. "An overview on the nutrition transition and its health implications: The Bellagio Meeting." *Public Health Nutrition* 5 (1A):93–103.

Popkin, Barry M. 1994. "The nutrition Transition in low-income countries: An emerging crisis." *Nutrition Reviews* 52 (9):285–298. doi: 10.1111/j.1753-4887.1994.tb01460.x.

Popkin, Barry M. 2004. "The nutrition transition: An overview of world patterns of change." *Nutrition Reviews* 62:S140–S143. doi: 10.1111/j.1753-4887.2004.tb00084.x.

Popkin, Barry M. 2012. "The nutrition transition is speeding up: A global perspective." In *Nutritional Health*, edited by Norman J. Temple, Ted Wilson, and Jr David R. Jacobs, 85–99. Humana Press.

Popkin, Barry M. 2015. "Nutrition transition and the global diabetes epidemic." *Current Diabetes Reports* 15 (9):1–8.

Popkin, Barry M. 2017. "Relationship between shifts in food system dynamics and acceleration of the global nutrition transition." *Nutrition Reviews* 75 (2):73–82.

Popkin, B. M., G. Keyou, F. Zhai, X. Guo, H. Ma, and N. Zohoori. 1993. "The nutrition transition in China: A cross-sectional analysis." *European Journal of Clinical Nutrition* 47 (5):333–346.

Popkin, Barry M., Linda S. Adair, and Shu Wen Ng. 2012. "Global nutrition transition and the pandemic of obesity in developing countries." *Nutrition Reviews* 70 (1):3–21. doi: 10.1111/j.1753-4887.2011.00456.x.

Popkin, B.M., and T. Reardon. 2018. "Obesity and the food system transformation in Latin America." *Obesity Reviews* 19 (8):1028–1064.

Powell, B., A. Ouarghidi, T. Johns, M. Ibn Tattou, and P. Eyzaguirre. 2014. "Wild leafy vegetable use and knowledge across multiple sites in Morocco: A case study for transmission of local knowledge?" *Journal of Ethnobiology and Ethnomedicine* 10:11. doi: 10.1186/1746-4269-10-34.

Power, Madeleine, Eleonora Uphoff, Brian Kelly, and Kate E Pickett. 2017. "Food insecurity and mental health: An analysis of routine primary care data of pregnant women in the Born in Bradford cohort." *Journal of Epidemiol Community Health* 71 (4):324–328.

Pratt, Jeff. 2007. "Food values the local and the authentic." *Critique of Anthropology* 27 (3):285–300.

Preston-Werner, Theresa. 2009. “Gallo Pinto: Tradition, memory, and identity in Costa Rican foodways.” *Journal of American Folklore* 11–27.

Punch, Samantha, Ian McIntosh, and Ruth Emond. 2010. “Children’s food practices in families and institutions.” *Children's Geographies* 8 (3):227–232.

Quesada, Dayana, and Gómez, Georgina 2018. Consumo de panes en la población urbana costarricense. In *Estudio Latinoamérica y Nutrición y Salud.* ILSI Mesoamérica.

Rayner, Geof, Corinna Hawkes, Tim Lang, and Walden Bello. 2006. “Trade liberalization and the diet transition: A public health response.” *Health Promotion International* 21 (suppl 1):67–74.

Reardon, Thomas, C. Peter Timmer, Christopher B. Barrett, and Julio Berdegué. 2003. “The rise of supermarkets in Africa, Asia, and Latin America.” *American Journal of Agricultural Economics* 85 (5):1140–1146.

Reardon, Thomas, C. Peter Timmer, and Julio A. Berdegué. 2005. “Supermarket expansion in Latin America and Asia.” *New Directions in Global Food Markets,* 47–61.

Reserve, Monteverde Cloud Forest Biological. n.d. “Biodiversity.” http://www.reservamonteverde.com/biodiversity.html.

Rhee, Jinnie J., Josiemer Mattei, and Hannia Campos 2012. “Association between commercial and traditional sugar-sweetened beverages and measures of adiposity in Costa Rica.” *Public Health Nutrition* 15 (8).

Ritchie, Brent W., Chris Cooper, Christopher P. Cooper, and Neil Carr. 2003. *Managing Educational Tourism. [electronic resource], Aspects of Tourism: 10.* Clevedon; Buffalo, NY: Channel View Publications.

Ritchie, Lorrene D., and Janet C. King. 2008. “Nutrient recommendations and dietary guidelines for pregnant women.” In *Handbook of Nutrition and Pregnancy*, 3–25. Springer.

Rivera, Juan A., Simon Barquera, Teresa Gonzalez-Cossio, Gustavo Olaiz, and Jaime Sepulveda. 2004. “Nutrition transition in Mexico and in other Latin American countries.” *Nutrition Reviews* 62 (suppl 2):S149–S157.

Rivers-Moore, Megan. 2016. *Gringo Gulch: Sex, Tourism, and Social Mobility in Costa Rica.* University of Chicago Press.

Robinson, William I. 1998. “(Mal) Development in Central America: Globalization and social change.” *Development and Change* 29 (3):467–497.

Rockwell, Marvin. 2015. “History of the quakers.”

Romero-Daza, Nancy, and Andrea Freidus. 2008. “Female tourists, casual sex, and HIV risk in Costa Rica.” *Qualitative Sociology* 31 (2):169–187. doi: 10.1007/s11133-008-9096-y.

Roos, Gun. 2002. “Our bodies are made of pizza—food and embodiment among children in Kentucky.” *Ecology of Food and Nutrition* 41 (1):1–19. doi: 10.1080/03670240212534.

Rose, Donald, and Victor Oliveira. 1997. “Nutrient intakes of individuals from food-insufficient households in the United States.” *American Journal of Public Health* 87 (12):1956–1961.

Rose, Donald Diego. 2008. “Interventions to reduce household food insecurity: A synthesis of current concepts and approaches for Latin America.” *Revista de Nutrição* 21:159s–173s.

Roseboom, Tessa J., Jan H.P. Van Der Meulen, Anita C.J. Ravelli, Clive Osmond, David J.P. Barker, and Otto P. Bleker. 2001. "Effects of prenatal exposure to the Dutch famine on adult disease in later life: An overview." *Twin Research* 4 (5):293–298.

Ruiz, Ernesto. 2014. "Growing children: The relationship between food insecurity and child growth and development." PhD, University of South Florida.

Ruiz, Ernesto, David A. Himmelgreen, Nancy Romero Daza, and Jenny Peña. 2014. "Using a biocultural approach to examine food insecurity in the context of economic transformations in Rural Costa Rica." *Annals of Anthropological Practice* 38 (2):232–249.

Saenz, Luis. 2015. "Introduction to Monteverde ancient human population history."

Sahlins, Marshall D. 1981. *Historical Metaphors and Mythical Realities: Structure in the Early History of the Sandwich Islands Kingdom.* University of Michigan Press.

Sahoo, Subarnalata, and Basumati Panda. 2005. "Dietary pattern of expectant mothers: A study from the rural area of Balasore District, Orissa." *Journal of Human Ecology* 17 (4):301–305.

Salud, Ministerio de. 2015. "Meeting of CEGIREH."

Santana, E., and B. G. Milligan. 1984. "Behavior of Toucanets, Bellbirds, and Quetzals feeding on Lauraceous Fruits." *Biotropica* 16 (2):152–154.

Sarlio-Lähteenkorva, Sirpa, and Eero Lahelma. 2001. "Food insecurity is associated with past and present economic disadvantage and body mass index." *The Journal of nutrition* 131 (11):2880–2884.

Schmeer, Kammi K., Barbara A. Piperata, Andrés Herrera Rodríguez, Virgilio Mariano Salazar Torres, and Francisco José Centeno Cárdenas. 2015. "Maternal resources and household food security: Evidence from Nicaragua." *Public Health Nutrition* 18 (16):2915–2924.

Schmidhuber, Joseph, and Prakash Shetty. 2005. "Nutrition transition, obesity and noncommunicable diseases: Drivers, outlook and concerns." *SCN News* 29:13–19.

Scrimshaw, Carlos Muñoz, and S. Nevin, eds. 1995. *The Nutrition and Health Transition of Democratic Costa Rica.* Boston: International Foundation for Developing Countries.

Seckler, David. 1980. "'Malnutrition': An intellectual Odyssey." *Western Journal of Agricultural Economics* 5 (2):219–227.

Shepard, G., D. Arora, and A. Lampman. 2008. "The grace of the flood: Classification and use of wild mushrooms among the highland Maya of Chiapas." *Economic Botany* 62 (3):437–470. doi: 10.1007/s12231-008-9044-5.

Shin, D., K. W. Lee, and W. O. Song. 2015. "Dietary patterns during pregnancy are associated with risk of gestational Diabetes Mellitus." *Nutrients* 7 (11):9369–9382. doi: 10.3390/nu7115472.

Shusterman, Richard. 1999. *Bourdieu: A Critical Reader*, *Critical Readers*. Oxford; Malden, MA: Blackwell, 1999.

Simkhada, B., M. A. Porter, and E. R. van Teijlingen. 2010. "The role of mothers-in-law in antenatal care decision-making in Nepal: A qualitative study." *BMC Pregnancy and Childbirth* 10:10. doi: 10.1186/1471-2393-10-34.

Singer, Merrill. 1998. "The development of critical medical anthropology: Implications for biological anthropology." *Building a New Biocultural Synthesis:*

Politicaleconomic Perspectives on Human Biology, edited by A.H. Goodman and T.L. Leatherman, 93–123.

Singer, Merrill. 2001. "Toward a bio-cultural and political economic integration of alcohol, tobacco and drug studies in the coming century." *Social Science & Medicine* 53 (2):199–213.

Singer, Merill, and Scott Clair. 2003. "Syndemics and public health: Reconceptualizing disease in bio-social context." *Medical anthropology quarterly* 17 (4):423–441.

Smith, Gavin A., and R. Brooke Thomas. 1998. "What could be: Biocultural anthropology for the next generation." In *Building a New Biocultural Synthesis: Political-Economic Perspectives on Human Biology*, edited by Alan H. Goodman and Thomas L. Leatherman, 451–474. Ann Arbor: University of Michigan Press.

Snow, B. K. 1977. "Territorial behavior and courtship of Male 3-Wattled bellbird." *Auk* 94 (4):623–645.

Sobo, Elisa J. 2011. "Medical anthropology in disciplinary context: Definitional struggles and key debates (or answering the Cri Du Coeur)." *A Companion to Medical Anthropology*, 7–28.

Society, DOHaD. 2013. "Home." accessed November 20, 2013. http://www.mrc.soton.ac.uk/dohad/index.asp.

Southerton, Dale. 2013. "Habits, routines and temporalities of consumption: From individual behaviours to the reproduction of everyday practices." *Time & Society* 22 (3):335–355.

Stini, William A. 1995. "Osteoporosis in biocultural perspective." *Annual Review of Anthropology* 24: 397–421.

Stocker, Karen. 2013. *Tourism and Cultural Change in Costa Rica: Pitfalls and Possibilities*. Lexington Books.

Stuart-Macadam, Patricia, and Katherine A Dettwyler. 1995. "Breastfeeding." In *Biocultural Perspectives,* New York.

Sychareun, V., V. Hansana, V. Somphet, S. Xayavong, A. Phengsavanh, and R. Popenoe. 2012. "Reasons rural Laotians choose home deliveries over delivery at health facilities: A qualitative study." *BMC Pregnancy and Childbirth* 12:10. doi: 10.1186/1471-2393-12-86.

Tarasuk, Valerie S., and George H. Beaton. 1999. "Women's dietary intakes in the context of household food insecurity." *The Journal of Nutrition* 129 (3):672–679.

Tessier, Sophie, and Mariette Gerber. 2005. "Factors determining the nutrition transition in two Mediterranean islands: Sardinia and Malta." *Public Health Nutrition* 8 (08):1286–1292.

Thow, Anne Marie. 2009. "Trade liberalisation and the nutrition transition: Mapping the pathways for public health nutritionists." *Public Health Nutrition* 12 (11):2150–2158.

Thow, Anne Marie, and Corinna Hawkes. 2009. "The implications of trade liberalization for diet and health: A case study from Central America." *Globalization and Health* 5 (5):1–11.

Tijerina Saenz, Alexandra, Erik Ramirez Lopez, Victor Manuel Meneses Valderrama, and Nancy Edith Martinez Garza. 2014. "Intakes of energy and macronutrients in pregnant women in the northeast of Mexico." *Archivos latinoamericanos de nutrición* 64 (3):174–81.

Tours, Costa Rica Study. 2013. "Monteverde cheese factory tour." http://monteverdecheesefactory.com/.

Trabace, L., P. Tucci, L. Ciuffreda, M. Matteo, F. Fortunato, P. Campolongo, V. Trezza, and V. Cuomo. 2015. "'Natural' relief of pregnancy-related symptoms and neonatal outcomes: Above all do no harm." *Journal of Ethnopharmacology* 174:396–402. doi: 10.1016/j.jep.2015.08.046.

Twine, Richard. 2015. "Understanding snacking through a practice theory lens." *Sociology of Health & Illness* 37 (8):1270–1284.

Uauy, Ricardo, and Carlos Augusto Monteiro. 2004. "The challenge of improving food and nutrition in Latin America." *Food & Nutrition Bulletin* 25 (2):175–182.

Ulijaszek, Stanley J, and Hayley Lofink. 2006. "Obesity in biocultural perspective." *Annual Review of Anthropology*. 35:337–360.

USDA. 2015. "Food Tracker."

Valverde, Carlos Muñoz, and José Manuel. 1995. "Problems and challenges of the health sector during the 1980s." In *The Nutrition and Health Transition of Democratic Costa Rica*, edited by Carlos Muñoz and Nevin S. Scrimshaw. Boston: International Foundation for Developing Countries.

Van Zee, Erynee, Corbyn Cools, Shirley Castillo, and Kristin Hall. 2014. Greywater management in the Monteverde Zone: Perceptions, challenges, and solutions. In *Community Health 2014*. Monteverde: University of South Florida and the Monteverde Institute.

Vivanco, Luis A. 2006. *Green Encounters: Shaping and Contesting Environmentalism in Rural Costa Rica*. Vol. 3. Berghahn Books.

Wadsworth. 2011. *Diet Analysis Plus (10th edition)*. Cengage.

Waibel, Leo. 1939. "White settlement in Costa Rica." *Geographical Review* 29 (4):529–560.

Wallace, L.M., K.E. Brown, and S. Hilton. 2014. "Planning for, implementing and assessing the impact of health promotion and behaviour change interventions: A way forward for health psychologists." *Health psychology Review* 8 (1):8–33.

Wang, Caroline C. 1999. "Photovoice: A participatory action research strategy applied to women's health." *Journal of Women's health* 8 (2):185–192.

Warf, Barney. 2010. "Do you know the way to San José? Medical tourism in Costa Rica." *Journal of Latin American Geography* 9 (1):51–66.

Warr, Peter. 2014. "Food insecurity and its determinants." *Australian Journal of Agricultural and Resource Economics* 58 (4):519–537.

Watkins, Lara Louise. 2009. *Beyond Ethnicity as Risk Factor: Biocultural Context and Correlates of Type 2 Diabetes in a Cambodian American Community*. University of Connecticut.

Webber, Laura, Fanny Kilpi, Tim Marsh, Ketevan Rtveladze, Martin Brown, and Klim McPherson. 2012. "High rates of obesity and non-communicable diseases predicted across Latin America." *PloS One* 7 (8):e39589.

Weber, Karin. 2001. "Outdoor adventure tourism: A review of research approaches." *Annals of Tourism Research* 28 (2):360–377. doi: http://dx.doi.org/10.1016/S0160-7383(00)00051-7.

Weijzen, Pascalle LG, Cees de Graaf, and Garmt B Dijksterhuis. 2009. "Predictors of the consistency between healthy snack choice intentions and actual behaviour." *Food Quality and Preference* 20 (2):110–119.

Weller, Susan C., and A. Kimball Romney. 1988. *Systematic Data Collection [electronic resource], Qualitative Research Methods.* Vol. 10. Newbury Park, CA; London: SAGE, c1988.

Whitaker, Robert C., Shannon M. Phillips, and Sean M. Orzol. 2006. "Food insecurity and the risks of depression and anxiety in mothers and behavior problems in their preschool-aged children." *Pediatrics* 118 (3):e859–e868.

White, Darcy, Michelle Dynes, Marcie Rubardt, Koman Sissoko, and Rob Stephenson. 2013. "The influence of intrafamilial power on maternal health care in Mali: Perspectives of women, men and mothers-in-law." *International Perspectives on Sexual and Reproductive Health.* 58–68.

WHO. 2011. *Costa Rica: NCD Country Profiles.*

WHO. 2016. *Costa Rica: Diabetes Country Profile.*

WHO. 2016. "Q&A on the carcinogenicity of the consumption of red meat and processed meat." accessed February 16, 2016. http://www.who.int/features/qa/cancer-red-meat/en/.

WHO. 2016a. "Food security." World Health Organization, accessed November 18, 2013. http://www.who.int/trade/glossary/story028/en/.

WHO. 2018. *The State of Food Security and Nutrition in the World 2018: Building Climate Resilience for Food Security and Nutrition.* World Health Organization and Food & Agriculture Org.

Wiley, Andrea S. 1992. "Adaptation and the biocultural paradigm in medical anthropology: A critical review." *Medical Anthropology Quarterly* 6 (3):216–236.

Wiley, Andrea S., and Jennifer M. Cullin. 2016. "What do anthropologists mean when they use the term biocultural?" *American Anthropologist* 118 (3):554–569.

Wilk, Richard R. 1999. "'Real Belizean Food': Building local identity in the transnational Caribbean." *American Anthropologist* 101 (2):244–255. doi: 10.2307/683199.

Wilson, Tamar Diana. 2008. "Introduction: The impacts of tourism in Latin America." *Latin American Perspectives* 35 (3):3–20. doi: 10.2307/27648094.

Young, Sera, Barnabas Natamba, Flavia Luwedde, Dorcas Nyafwono, Ben Okia, Beth Osterbauer, Paul Natureeba, Lynn Johnson, Chloe Michel, and Amy Zheng. 2014. "'I have remained strong because of that food': Acceptability and use of lipid-based nutrient supplements among pregnant HIV-infected Ugandan women receiving combination antiretroviral therapy." *AIDS and Behavior*, 1–13.

Zuckerman, Molly K., and Debra L. Martin. 2016. *New Directions in Biocultural Anthropology.* John Wiley & Sons.

Zúniga, Joaquín. 2009. *Sun and Shadows [electronic resource]: The Downside of Tourism in Central America*, by Joaquín Zúniga, Filmakers library online. New York, NY: Filmakers Library, 2009. Videorecording.

Index

Page references for figures are italicized

About the Author

Allison R. Cantor is a medical anthropologist. She is a research affiliate at the Monteverde Institute and adjunct assistant professor at New Mexico State University. Allison is also an instructor for the Council on International Education Exchange.

www.ingramcontent.com/pod-product-compliance
Ingram Content Group UK Ltd.
Pitfield, Milton Keynes, MK11 3LW, UK
UKHW021027041026
15470UKWH00013B/71

9 781793 604255